Keto Diet for Women Over 50

The Scientifically Proven Method for Burning Excess Fat, with Easy Exercises and a Low Carb Meal Plan for a Keto Lifestyle

By

Sasha Taylor

TABLE OF CONTENTS

INTRODUCTION

The ketogenic diet (KD) is defined as a diet high in lipids, adequate in proteins, and low in carbohydrates that cause ketosis which minimizes potential Side effects on growth.

There are biblical references regarding the use of fasting as a treatment for a convulsive picture. The first modern use of fasting as a treatment of the Epilepsy goes back to 1911; Guelpa and Marie treat 20 patients of infantile age and adults without specifying more details. It can be said that fasting was a precursor to the use of DC as a treatment in epilepsy.

In 1921, Woodyatt and Wilder demonstrated the appearance of acetone and hydroxybutyric acid in fasting subjects, which improved epileptic seizures. This encouraged Peterman to create what is now known as a ketogenic diet, for which it indicates that should be individualized and with the requirement of close monitoring of the patients, and with which beneficial effects on behavior and development are achieved cognitive. These studies were followed at Harvard by Talbot, and at the Mayo Clinic by MacQuarrie and Keith.

DC had already been mentioned as a tool to control

epileptic seizures in many texts, but it was in 1972 when Livingston reported the result of the diet administered to 1,000 children with epilepsy, proving that 52% of them had obtained complete control of the crises and that in 27% there was a large improvement.

In 1971, P. Huttenlocher introduced medium-chain triglycerides (TCM) in the preparation of the diets. From 1970 to 2000, the use of KD decreased in a considerable way; Only two publications per year appear with this reference.

Currently, KD is used in more than 50 countries, it is initially indicated in the deficit of GLUT-1 and in the deficit of pyruvate dehydrogenase, and should be considered as a first-line treatment in infantile spasms, myoclonic seizures, tuberous sclerosis, myoclonic-asthmatic epilepsy (Doose's syndrome), in Dravet syndrome, in Rett syndrome and in Lennox-Gastaut syndrome, which are refractory to antiepileptic medication. However, it should not be a treatment of the first choice in other convulsive syndromes; you must have into account when at least two modern anticonvulsant drugs have failed.

Finally, it is interesting to know the position of the Charlie Foundation in 2009:

"The KD has been documented in a consistent way regarding the efficacy of the treatment of epilepsy in hundreds of children since 1924. In the last 15 years, it verifies these results in about 750 reviews, they have published their implementation and its scientific mechanisms. There are two large communications which have included 44 reviews concerning more than a hundred children who received a KD as a treatment, confirming that at least 50% or more improved their convulsive crisis."

CHAPTER 1

WHAT IS THE KETO OR KETOGENIC DIET?

The ketogenic diet is a diet rich in lipids particularly fashionable for some years. However, it has been used for almost a hundred years to treat certain pathologies, including epilepsy. This diet aims to significantly reduce the consumption of carbohydrates in favor of lipids to cause a state of ketosis. Beyond the important weight loss, it would have many health benefits.

What Is The ketogenic Diet?

Both in the social and sporting fields, the ketogenic diet is a fast, safe and effective diet where you can triple the weight loss compared to a hypocaloric diet (low in calories) which is the most common diet we recommend. nutriólogos, in addition to reach our goal quickly during this transition will not present physiological hunger, as you read "you will not be hungry" this is achieved through the induction to a controlled ketosis, in a clinical aspect this means that the specialist will come down the load on the consumption of carbohydrates to less than 50 grams per day and give constant doses of protein, but be careful not any protein,must be a protein of high biological value this means that it contains all the essential amino acids that our body needs and that even some of them cannot produce on their own, and on the contrary you will have a state of well-being throughout the day.

Today there are different presentations of high biological value protein such as bars, soups, cakes, crepes, cookies, snacks, juices, etc. all of high-value protein, on the other hand, as in any diet hydration will be of utmost importance, it is advisable to take at least 2 liters of water, this can be controlled by counting the water glasses that are taken throughout the day or well always bring with us a thermos or a bottle of water that in addition to helping us reach the goal of water consumption, we will be collaborating with the conservation of the environment. An important point of the ketogenic diet will be to be supplemented with vitamins and minerals. The specialist is the only one who can recommend us the one that best suits our needs.

During this type of diet, the consumption of cereals, fruits, dairy products, cheeses, butters, among many other foods that should be indicated in the clinical or nutritional consultation will be limited only for a specific time, this does not mean that these foods are not allowed to be bad or should not be consumed, it is simply that being in a process of reduction of carbohydrates should be added gradually along with dietary reeducation guidelines dictated by the specialist this means that in addition to losing weight quickly our specialist in health we will be taught to eat healthily so that we can maintain this lost weight for a long time.

This gradual introduction of the different food groups will help our body to learn correctly how to metabolize all macronutrients such as proteins, fats and carbohydrates so that our body does not store them in the form of fat and we do not recover the lost weight.

The 4 Types Of A Ketogenic Diet

A strict ketogenic diet is extremely difficult to maintain. Since carbon forms all the organic life around us, it is impossible to avoid completely eating at least some carbohydrates during the day. In addition, carbohydrates are useful for muscle activity. This is why there are transient forms of the keto diet: those that aim to help the person reduce the number of carbohydrates while remaining appetizing. The key here is to experiment and find what works better for you rather than blindly following pre-made formulas.

The standard ketogenic diet (SKD). This form of ketogenic diet simply aims to reduce carbohydrate intake to 30g a day and is intended for people who do not exercise on a regular basis.

The targeted ketogenic diet (TKD). If you eat carbs just before and after exercise, you do TKD. It's that simple — ideal for people who exercise moderately during the day.

Ketogenic Cyclic Regime (CKD). This is where we become serious. CKD involves loading a lot of carbohydrates at specific times and then exercising to spend everything. Ideal for people who have serious training regimes or who are professional athletes.

High protein ketogenic diet (HPKD). A Regular ketogenic diet that minimizes carbohydrates and proteins. The HPKD aims to increase muscle mass through a diet of 60% fat, 35-40% protein, and 0-5% carbohydrates.

CHAPTER 2

BENEFITS OF THE KETOGENIC DIET

When we use mainly carbohydrates as an energy source, our cells burn the glucose they contain, since carbohydrates are only long chains of different types of sugars. Sugar is also a great source of energy, but unlike that produced by fats, glucose as an energy source is expensive because in the process of combustion of glucose, or glycolysis, many of the so-called " free radicals," substances harmful to us that are behind diseases such as cancer, chronic inflammation or premature aging.

Ketone bodies and fats are more efficient at metabolizing cells and producing much less "waste."

1. Insulin control

Insulin is a hormone that is produced in the pancreas and has the function of transporting glucose into the cell and, in that way, regulate its levels in the blood. In this modern world in which we live, in which we eat continuously and ingest high levels of carbohydrates, the body is forced to constantly produce this hormone to introduce the glucose into the cells and decrease those constants peaks in blood.

When we ingest large amounts of sugars, fruit, flours, or other foods rich in carbohydrates, the pancreas works tirelessly on insulin production. When these carbohydrates are also high glycemic index and cause sudden rises in blood sugar, glucose peaks force the pancreas to work at full capacity to generate sufficient amounts of insulin, which can exhaust it.

That is why diets high in carbohydrates, and especially high glycemic index carbohydrates, are associated with the development of insulin resistance and diabetes.

2. Loss of body fat

A ketogenic diet stabilizes the hormones that regulate the appetite, prioritizes the metabolic processes that accelerate the combustion of fats, and increases the sensation of satiety.

By decreasing body fat, the relative percentage of muscle mass with respect to our weight increases. This not only has aesthetic repercussions, certainly not negligible, but also for our health, since it accelerates the virtuous circle of a greater sensitivity to insulin (which was already initiated by the fact of limiting the glucose peaks), improves the function of Most organs increase osteoarticular mobility and limit the risk of joint damage thanks to the protective reinforcement that the musculature for the skeleton supposes.

3. Anti-aging effect

In a general way, a high caloric intake ages us. When we constantly eat, as most Western societies do, carbohydrates and processed foods, this roller coaster of blood sugar are followed, as we have seen above, followed by an insulin surge to compensate for it with the subsequent sudden descent of glucose that leaves us weak and hungry. In this whole process, we will not only gain fat, but we are also accelerating our metabolism, causing our cells to generate more free radicals and divide more quickly than they would with a more moderate intake of food.

In this scenario of high intake of food in general and carbohydrates in particular, the body is less efficient when it comes to repair and recycle existing cells, and ends up choosing to manufacture new ones. This mechanism can accelerate the aging process because, during the manufacture of new cells, more toxic waste and waste products are produced than when it is simply dedicated to repairing existing ones.

With a ketogenic diet, we tend to eat less, with a positive domino effect on longevity, minimization of metabolic damage and physical appearance.

Eating keto usually produces a natural reduction in appetite. Although sometimes and depending on the person and its objectives can become a problem, it generally has a very positive effect on the regulation of caloric intake.

4. Optimization of the immune system

A body adapted to burn fat and ketone bodies increases the production of antioxidant enzymes, such as cattail or glutathione, which have a powerful and broad effect on the body. These antioxidant enzymes help to reduce inflammation and oxidative stress generated by poor nutritional habits, intense physical exercise, or simply the minimal damage caused by being alive, breathing and burning calories.

In this way, the ketogenic diet improves our immune system significantly, delaying aging, minimizing neuronal damage, and reducing the possibility of developing diseases and infections. We will also look more beautiful. These enzymes have an especially powerful effect in keeping our skin young and healthy, maintaining its elasticity and protecting it from damage caused by the environment, the sun and other agents.

5. Cognitive improvement

Ketone bodies easily cross the barrier between the tiny blood vessels and the brain and are a very efficient source of energy for the nervous system, optimizing the enzymatic function and the synthesis of neurotransmitters, which increase your ability to connect neuronal cells. That is why ketosis and a ketogenic diet reduce mental fatigue and increase the ability to concentrate.

It has also been proven that when your brain uses ketone bodies as an energy source, it suffers less damage in the long term: in a certain way, it protects it from degenerative diseases associated with cognitive worsening, such as lack of concentration, memory loss or senile diseases.

6. Protection against tumors and cancer

Tumor cells proliferate at a much higher rate than healthy cells in a glucose-rich environment, consuming up to 200 times more sugars. This is what is known as the Warburg Effect, by the scientist Otto Warburg, who discovered this metabolic mechanism in cancer cells over one hundred years ago.

Being in ketosis limits the growth of tumor cells since in most cases, they cannot be nourished by ketone bodies. When we eat a diet high in healthy fats and limit carbohydrates, we are limiting the proliferation of tumor cells.

It has long been used fasting and caloric restriction to reduce the availability of glucose tumor cells and can be a complement to traditional treatments used to fight cancer.

Unlike glucose, which can be used in the synthesis of energy in the absence of oxygen (is what is called "anaerobic glycolysis"), ketones require oxygen to be transformed into energy, and this occurs in a part of the cell called mitochondria. One of the characteristics of tumor cells is that they have damaged their mitochondrial function, so most of them cannot use ketone bodies but glucose, which does not require this function.

7. Improvement in metabolism

The ketones are not just a source of clean, efficient energy for our cells, but also act as an element that initiates anti-inflammatory and positively regulate metabolism. This effect is very powerful, and it has an effect on the activation or not of certain genes, that is, it has an epigenetic impact.

By reducing oxidative stress, using these bodies as a fuel instead of sugar is especially relevant in improving the cardiovascular system, because the heart and the complex vascular system are especially sensitive to the oxidative effects of high-carbohydrate diets.

Ketone bodies also seem to be especially beneficial for our mitochondria, that part of the cell that generates energy and is so important for our health. As we have seen, we can use glucose as fuel without the need for oxygen or the intervention of the mitochondria in the process, so the continued consumption of carbohydrates can, in a certain way, atrophy our mitochondria, reducing their efficiency and impacting negatively in our metabolism.

8. Emotional and humor improvement

Addiction to carbohydrates not only leads to that roller coaster of physical weakness, hunger, and lack of concentration but also does the same with our emotional state and our mood. When your body is not adapted to use fats and depends on that constant glucose drug as an energy source, you need to eat very often and the process is perpetuated over time.

Resetting your metabolism and re-teaching you to also burn ketone bodies will free you from that dependence on glucose and stabilize your mood and your mood. Instead of going through life as on a roller coaster, it will be something like riding a bike through gentle hills; There will also be variations, of course, but they will be much less pronounced and the falls will not be so abrupt.

9. Improvement of physical performance

In endurance sports, the ability to burn fat as the intensity of the race increases is the cornerstone that differentiates faster runners from those who are not able to keep up with them.

In strength and power sports, not depending on glucose reduces inflammation, and optimizes the regulation of protein synthesis, which will allow you to train more intensively, reduce the risk of injury and recover faster.

The conventional theory of sports performance says that when we are doing a resistance exercise, for example, running an ultra-distance race, depending on certain variables, there may come a time when we run out of glucose in our system and are unable to continue. It's something that happens suddenly. The muscles do not respond, we feel extreme weakness and we are almost incapable of standing. It is what is popularly known as a "pajara," an acute state of hypoglycemia in which the muscles are literally unable to activate because they have run out of fuel.

The Theory of the Central Governor Question this explanation. In essence, it comes to say that it is the brain that sends the order to the muscles not to get going and that in reality, we still have enough energy in the cells to continue. The energy consumption has been such that the brain considers that, unless something very serious happens as a life-threatening situation, for example, the remaining energy must be saved. This theory of the Central Governor would be in contradiction with the classical theory that fatigue depends on the situation of the peripheral muscles. In fact, it has been seen that it is possible to "tap" the brain in situations in which hypoglycemia theoretically has us in that state of almost immobility, muscle pain and nausea and yet we are able to continue.

The question that is still being investigated is to what extent this "gap" appears before because of the widespread use of fuel as inefficient as carbohydrates in the world of endurance sports than what appears in athletes adapted to burn grease. In the coming years, studies that are currently underway will appear, which seem, a priori, to point in this direction.

Ketogenic Diet And Gene Expression

A high intake of sugar and poor quality carbohydrates not only makes us gain weight and increases the likelihood of developing autoimmune diseases, diabetes, and cardiovascular disease but also damages our DNA .

For decades, it was assumed that DNA was something immutable, something rigid that was transmitted from father to son, and that determined many factors of our life, from our eye color to our personality or our ability to solve arithmetic problems. However, in recent years, it has been seen that the type of life we lead also affects our DNA .

What does this mean? Imagine that a woman has what the press and the media call "the breast cancer gene." A healthy lifestyle and some vital habits that enhance their well-being are not going to make that gene disappear, but what they can achieve is that it is not expressed, that is, that it is there, but it is not "active."

Sugar, high glycemic index carbohydrates, processed foods, and poor quality fats favor the expression of genes that promote the disease. A diet rich in healthy fats, vegetables, and good quality proteins can help to silence those genes.

Not only this. We could say that a diet low in carbohydrates and processed foods rich in healthy fats activate the genes of "health," "energy," or "burn fat," improving our quality of life, our resistance to diseases and our longevity.

CHAPTER 3

CHANGES IN YOUR BODY AFTER 50

If you have passed thirty, you will have noticed: your body begins to change from that age. Unfortunately, it is not always easy to face these changes as something positive.

Throughout our trajectory, not only are our circumstances (work, family, couple) and the life we lead (schedules and customs) changed; There are also modifications in our interior. Some of these make it really difficult for us to keep fit or lose weight if that is our goal . Therefore, today we will see what those changes that occur in our bodies from the 50s are and how to deal with them.

Body Changes in 50

These are the changes that occur in your body after 50; the culprits of keeping fit is such a complex matter:

Decrease In Testosterone Levels

With the arrival of andropause, the hormone levels begin to be reduced gradually affecting the functioning of our body. And since testosterone is one of the main hormones responsible for muscle production and toning, once its levels decline, the performance of, for example, sports training, is diminished.

Of course, a decrease in testosterone can cause a significant loss of muscle mass.

If you think this may be happening to you, we invite you to check it out with this quick and simple test: Check your testosterone levels.

Metabolism Slowdown

From 40/50 years of age, our basal metabolism (minimum calories that the body requires and consumes to digest food, generate hormones, and other basic functions of the human body) is reduced. This means that, when at 20 years of age, a man of 1.90 and 80Kg of weight required a minimum of 2500Kcal, today he will not need more than 1500Kcal.

The problem is that, generally, at 50, we want to continue eating the same thing we ate before, which gives the body an excess of calories that we do not spend and that inevitably translates into weight gain.

Reduction Of Muscle Mass And Increased Fat

As we told you at the beginning, the decrease in testosterone levels causes a reduction in muscle mass. In parallel, fat increases.

In this way, the metabolism decreases even more since we have a greater amount of fat and less active tissue (muscle, which in turn is the one that burns the most calories).

How To Keep Body Changes At 50

At this point, you probably think that, after 50, it is almost impossible to maintain a healthy weight. But the reality is that the effects of age and body changes of 50 can be mitigated and even avoided completely if we follow some guidelines.

1. Take care of your diet

Following a diet rich in nutrients, antioxidants, and vitamins can help reduce the effects of time and severity.

2. Train your body

Performing exercises on a regular basis, working strength, and activating the muscles can be a great way to reverse body changes from a certain age. In addition, it has been shown that performing physical exercise contributes to the production of testosterone in a natural way. Of course, if you are being treated for a hormonal deficit level, the sport will also be a great ally when it comes to seeing positive results.

3. Try To Have A Proper Rest

Did you know that high-stress levels, in addition to causing anxiety, can make you fat? Therefore, among other reasons, getting a restful break is a key point in maintaining physical and mental fitness at any age.

4. Visit A Health Professional

Although you can find a lot of information on the Internet, the best thing you can do for your health is to visit a medical professional who performs some basic tests (the complete analysis, biometrics, electrocardiogram, etc.) and can assess your state as a whole before prescribing yourself No type of treatment.

On The Other Hand

Probably, one of the great reasons why the woman who is in her fifties begins to notice real changes, both physical and emotional, is mainly due to the arrival of menopause. But what are the most frequent symptoms that identify menopause?

Menopause occurs because the woman's ovaries stop producing progesterone. The woman, when she reaches menopause, therefore, stops having a menstrual period for a year, although changes and symptoms may begin several years earlier. Menopause usually occurs, in addition, between 45 and 55 years, but most often, it appears around fifty, and hence many changes appear and women notice them at this age.

For the vast majority, the menstrual periods will stop slowly over time, and during this period, the periods may be happening with a narrower or wider interval. These variations may last between one and three years, approximately, but it will not be until the woman has not been a full year without having the period when menopause really takes place. Also, the woman can discover it by the symptoms that will appear. Do you know which are the most common?

The most common menopause symptoms are usually hot flashes, mood swings, and sexual problems, although many others also appear quite common such as these:

- Irregular level of flow during menstruation and irregular menstrual periods during premenopause
- Depression, the feeling of sadness, nervousness, anxiety, and palpitations stronger than usual
- Hot flashes and extreme sensation of body heat that usually lasts several minutes
- Breast pain decreased sex drive and weight gain
- Severe headaches, migraines, insomnia, irritability
- Vaginal dryness and dry skin

And what to do to prevent such symptoms?

- Give up smoking
- Do not drink alcohol
- Respect sleep schedules
- Exercise

And for hot flashes?

You will have already realized that hot flashes are one of the most annoying symptoms of menopause and, therefore, it is inevitable that women want to avoid them by all means. But what can they do? Hot flashes are that sudden sensation of heat in the chest and face that extends to the rest of the body and can cause excessive sweating . It is true that the frequency of hot flashes can be variable. In fact, some women suffer all day and others every hour.

Hot flashes are also likely to occur at night . Nighttime hot flashes probably also affect sleep quality, and signs of fatigue, irritability, and insomnia appear. And yes, they are very annoying, but much more with the winter heaters and the air conditioners of the summer that can also make the situation worse and much, so here are some tricks:

- One of the best ways to avoid hot flashes is to always dress in layers . So, if you are cold or hot, you can take off the odd layer of clothing without any difficulty.
- Avoiding large and overly copious meals is also a way to reduce the recurrence of hot flashes.
- Try not to consume drinks that are too cold or too hot, such as tea or infusions, since the thermal contrast with the body can cause the temperature to rise.
- use cold cloths. The idea of lowering body temperature thanks to skin contact with a cold cloth is great. In

this way, the feeling of heat will be drastically reduced.

- eliminate tobacco. Remember that tobacco can also eliminate the intensity of hot flashes because nicotine directly affects the central nervous system and causes changes in hormone secretion.

What else changes occur?

For many women, turning 50 is like riding a roller coaster, but without a belt (or that is at least what Sill Shaw Ruddock claimed, in his book "The Second Half of your life") in which he also refers to Menopause as that time of hormones that have regulated everything and begin to beat in retreat causing all those symptoms that we mentioned before such as anxiety, depression, insomnia, palpitations and even the desire to cry .

And yes, these are the changes of a lifetime. However, what will be a little more complicated to deal with will be the situation in which the 50-year-old woman is currently and which, of course, she did not face before. Why? Well, simply because formerly when the woman crossed the threshold of fifty children were already studying at the university, and even some of them had become independent or married. And now what happens?

Now things are quite different from what they were before because, with the delay of motherhood, the number of women around fifty who now have teenage children is quite high. This means, therefore, that they have to be dealing with all the changes in their bodies and in their minds and also with those of their teenage children with their revolutionized hormones. The calm, therefore, that women had before, now no longer have it.

However, the problem is not only there because, as the author affirms, "although emotions constitute a good turning point with the arrival of the fifties, it also is not at all the only change to pay attention to ." With the arrival of menopause, the skin gradually loses its thickness and becomes rougher and dehydrated especially as a result of the thinning of its increasingly dry and dry layers, and it is when women begin to discover that sagging has entered their lives, and there is a small transformation of their physiognomy, their contours have blurred and, in addition, their hair is increasingly dry and thin as a result of the disappearance of estrogens.

At this age, sexuality is also immersed because, with the arrival of menopause, the fall of estrogen causes a series of effects on the woman's organism that can end up turning the most intimate and passionate moments with the couple into true reluctance and even pain. In addition, as you get older, you also have to take into account that a wide range of diseases that can also affect sexual performance and interest begin to appear. Some of the most common are usually arthritis , blood pressure and heart disease .

And our great enemy, weight gain. With the arrival of menopause, problems related to food and weight are a focus of great importance and also of concern and discomfort for women, and what really happens is that women find a negative element in their weight when accepting their age and also the passage of time. Why? Simply because before the age of fifty, losing weight was much easier to do just by following a balanced diet and doing some exercise.

However, passing the fifties barrier makes this more complicated. Women at this age and with menopause feel more swollen and find it quite difficult to lose weight that perhaps with very little a few years ago, they did lose. The difficulty of losing weight also causes them to feel more insecure and irascible. In these cases, the best, no doubt, will be to go to an endocrine or a nutritionist to guide their steps and, above all, to prevent them from falling into large eating disorders.

And no, calm down because not everything is so negative. In fact, with this age and also with the arrival of menopause, there are many changes and very positive because women at this age have greater intellectual capacity . Remember that, with the passage of time, there are certain brain functions that are exacerbated, especially in those women who are and who remain really active. It is also a good time to completely abandon contraceptives if menstruation has come to an end because one can no longer get pregnant. And as many other women say, when you reach fifty , you really know who you are and, although it may seem strange at first, for many of them to break through the barrier of the fifties is the best time of life because they are already aware of what they want and do not want both personally and professionally.

CHAPTER 4

THE LONGEVITY GOAL

Some studies have proposed that weight gain around the waist is rather a factor in the aging process - which affects both sexes - rather than being caused by hormonal changes linked to menopause. However, other studies indicate that the reduction of estrogen (estradiol or E2) in the 50s modifies the energy needs and metabolism of women, changes the location of the accumulation of body fat from the hips to the abdomen and is associated with greater metabolic syndrome rate.

Dr. Wendy Kohrt of the University of Colorado, Denver, directs the IMAGE program (research on metabolism, age, sex and exercise) and studies the effects of menopause for more than 20 years. He has discovered that at 50, women's metabolism is reduced by about 50 calories a day and women experience more food cravings, less movement and more loss of muscle mass. Together, these four factors have a fairly large effect on the gradual increase in weight over time. However, Menopause itself has been little investigated over the years, taking into account the effect it has on the health and well-being of millions of women, an aspect that other commentators also a highlight.

There is a weight gain in the 50s - we all know it - but scientific research cannot explain it yet. It does not occur as universally as it is generally perceived. It is also not known very well why women who follow a ketogenic diet would have stagnations or even weight gain. We want to try to understand this better. "

Currently, the scientist is conducting a study in which ten overweight women, most 50, who follow a ketogenic diet, but whose weight loss has stalled early, will spend about five days in a monitored environment. During this time, your food and activity will be observed and recorded and your metabolism analyzed. Although similar studies have been done in the past, this is the first time that it has focused on women with weight loss stagnations on a low-carb and high-fat diet. Most of the other studies concluded that the root of the problem was excessive food consumption. We want to see what is happening with these women.

The results of the study will not be available for a few months. Until then, below, you can read the ten best tips from the experts to get you out of a stalemate. These apply to menopausal women in addition to anyone who experiences a stagnation in weight loss or is not having enough success with a ketogenic diet.

1. Do not eat too much protein

Do not eat too much protein: the number one cause of stagnation is excessive protein consumption. Women need less protein, and it is much easier for them to consume too much compared to men. If you and your husband are eating a loin of the same size, you are consuming too much protein. "

Consuming too much protein interferes with ketosis and fat burning and checking blood glucose after consuming protein to see if it goes up. "If it goes up, it means that a part of that protein has been converted into blood sugar. And that can delay you.

The researcher cares less about maintaining a moderate protein intake. But apart from it, the general advice of our group of experts is daily consumption of between 0.5 and 1.5 g of protein per kilo of body weight. A 70 kg (154 lb) woman would consume, then, no more than 105 g per day, and perhaps much less.

If you are not interested in counting grams, you might prefer to try a suggestion some researcher: make a "conscious week" and reform your feelings of hunger and satiety.

The problem and the challenge for all the people we consult, not only menopausal women, is that they don't know the feelings of hunger and satiety. They come to us after years and decades of following a diet low in fat and high in carbohydrates, so they have become accustomed to having a feeling of fullness only when they are already too full. Therefore, we need to retrain ourselves to understand that you should feel satisfied instead of full.

People always say: Wow, I have eaten a lot, and I feel so full and ugly. It is this feeling of being "full" that has become the usual… feeling uncomfortable after eating. So we have to retrain ourselves to understand that 'full enough' is how you should feel.

When a stalemate is causing difficulties, many people ask, Should I count calories again? No, no, no! Make a conscious week. The patient, in my opinion, should devote a week to the process. You have to spend a week because it takes time.

So, if you are used to breakfast with two eggs and two slices of bacon, during the conscious week, you would only bring one egg and a slice of bacon to the table. And you would eat them. Then you have to wait 20 minutes, and that's when the investment of time comes. After 20 minutes, you ask yourself, "Am I still hungry?

You have to give yourself time to learn if you are full or if you are still hungry, so you do this at every meal for a week. At some point, you will realize that you are eating an appropriate amount of food, too much food or too little food. After some meal you will realize I have eaten too much, I did not need that second egg or something similar. It is a way to do it without counting calories and based on the needs of your body and how you can connect with those needs.

Once you have adapted to burn fat, reduce the extra amount of fat you eat: one of the wonders of starting a ketogenic diet is to return to our bodies all the fat that we were deprived of for so long. But the ketogenic diet is not a white card to cram you with fat, experts note. If you want to lose weight, you need to burn your own body fat stores for energy, not consume all the energy you need in the form of dietary fat. So leave bulletproof coffees and grease pumps aside for now.

When people start the ketogenic diet for the first time after having consumed a lot of carbohydrates and being very dependent on glucose in the past, he tells them to eat unlimited amounts of healthy fats until they are fully adapted to the burning of grease. You will know that you are adapted to burn fat when you can spend a lot of time without eating.

However, once the fat burning capacity is optimized, the researcher reduces the fat consumption of some patients so that they begin to access and burn their fat deposits.

So if you are experiencing stagnation in weight loss, our experts recommend that you observe how much fat you are eating and if you can reduce this amount without harming the taste of your food or your feeling of satiety and without causing food cravings to return and the highs and lows of blood sugar. Do not deprive yourself of food, but be aware of excess fat for now. Some decided not to consume bulletproof coffee for a while.

It is easy to consume an excessive amount of fat in liquid form, especially whipping cream. Someone will come to the office and say they are stagnant in weight loss. We look at his diet and observe that he is drinking six cups of coffee, each with two tablespoons of whipping cream. Reducing the amount of cream this person consumes can get him out of the stalemate.

When you've reached your ideal weight, you can add all the fat you want again.

2. Intermittent fasting

Add intermittent fasting: once you adapt to fat burning, the hunger pangs decrease, and it becomes easy to spend long periods without eating. Many people stop having breakfast. Naturally, they just aren't hungry when they wake up. The number one norm of low carb eating is "eat when you are hungry and stop eating when you are satiated. So if you're not hungry, try fasting for 16 hours and have lunch and dinner within an 8-hour period, which is called fasting 16 and 8. Or, you can try to have dinner one night and fast until dinner the next day, so you fast for 24 hours.

For Ellen McCormick Martens, 71, of Houston, Texas, adding intermittent fasting and eating only between 11:00 am and 7:00 pm is what made it possible to overcome persistent stagnations in weight loss. "Using intermittent fasting, I have been able to maintain the loss of my excess weight for 1.5 years. It's really simple and easy to incorporate [a short fast] into a low-carb lifestyle.

The researcher advises not to do the same fast routine every day but to vary it by doing, for example, 16 and 8 a day and 24 hours of fasting the next day, followed by a day of eating regularly. It is because the body has a strong physiological impulse to seek homeostasis: the balance of energy. "When the body is exposed to constant stimulation, it will end up getting used to it.

However, the researcher advises being careful with long fasts that last several days. If you're skipping meals because you're not hungry by following a well-formulated diet low in carbohydrates and high in fat, that's fine. Instead, she worries about very long fasts that ignore hunger signals and that pose a risk of dangerous electrolyte and fluid imbalances, called the feedback syndrome, which can occur after long fasts that last multiple days, once Regular feeding resumes.

When people follow a ketogenic diet, they are often not hungry for 16, 24, and even 36 hours. These forms of fasting are safe and healthy. Remember: eat when you're hungry (don't eat when you're not) and stop eating when you're full.

3. Be careful that carbohydrates do not accumulate

You have to be attentive to the accumulation without realizing carbohydrates: if you have been eating low carb for a long time, they can start to sneak into your diet, especially in the form of sauces, condiments, fruits, and nuts. If the weight loss has stagnated, carefully examine what you are eating and again reduce carbohydrate intake to less than 20 g per day. Nuts such as cashews, almonds and pistachios are the easiest to consume in excess and contribute to stagnation in weight loss. One cup of pistachios, for example, contains 34 g of carbohydrates. Also, avoid for now any strategy of periodically consuming carbohydrates or trap foods.

In some people who are resistant to insulin, if they are in ketosis but consume only one meal with carbohydrates, this can stop ketosis for up to three weeks.

Keeping carbohydrate intake below 20 g maximizes weight loss and will give more control over hunger and cravings.

4. Eliminate alcohol consumption

Don't drink alcohol for now: many people love the fact that you can have a glass of dry wine (red or white) from time to time on a low carb or ketogenic diet. But if you have stagnated in weight loss, or are gaining weight, eliminate the consumption of all alcoholic beverages for now, until the weight loss begins again. Even having a couple of drinks a week can cause stagnation. I love having a glass of wine on Fridays after a hard week at work, but I will eliminate it for now.

5. Avoid sweeteners

Remove artificial sweeteners from your diet: if you have consumed sweeteners such as aspartame or sucralose as part of your low carb or keto diet, our experts recommend that you disengage them. Although there aren't many scientific studies, anecdotal information tells us that when people get rid of artificial sweeteners, they find it easier to lose weight. Stop using them as soon as possible.

6. Train with weights

No matter how fast you run, you cannot escape a bad diet. However, adding weight training will increase muscle mass and speed up your metabolism.

Lift weights No matter how fast you run, you cannot escape a bad diet. However, adding weight training to your low carb lifestyle will increase muscle mass and speed up your metabolism. The more muscle you accumulate, the better your insulin sensitivity will be, so any form of resistance effort you can exert on your muscles is great for weight loss. Weight training does not have to be excessive, doing 90 seconds twice a week may be enough, but note that the weight has to be enough so that, after doing about 10-15 repetitions, you can no longer. It is called lifting up to muscle failure. Only by reaching the absolute failure will you convince your body that you are not strong enough. Your body will not add more muscle if you don't give it the message that it needs more muscle. Striding, push-ups and other training methods that use bodyweight are as effective as using dumbbells or weight machines.

The researcher never mentions the subject of exercise as the first step in weight loss. He wants patients to focus first on food. But later, if things are not working as well as at the beginning and there is still an excess of weight to lose, I start talking about that word that begins with " E ": the exercise. However, I advise you to resume the activities that are fun for them. Exercise will help you break a deadlock. "

Intense exercise can sometimes create a false stagnation in weight loss. "If you exercise until your muscles ache, you are tearing a muscle, which is a good thing, it's how you increase muscle mass, causing tiny tears. But in order to deal with this, the body triggers a small inflammatory response that causes people to retain fluids. So after intense training, you can climb a couple of kilos overnight. It is not a real stalemate but a false one.

Be sure to give yourself rest days between high-intensity workouts so that the body has time to recover.

7. Get enough sleep

Sleeping well at night reduces stress and cortisol, the stress hormone that inhibits the loss of abdominal fat.

Sleep well at night: during menopause, many women observe a marked deterioration in sleep quality, often due to hot flashes and night sweats. Women who have stagnated in weight loss improve sleep quality. Sleeping well at night reduces stress and cortisol, the stress hormone that inhibits the loss of abdominal fat.

The best sleeping tips include:

- Sleep in a cool and darkroom.
- Wear earplugs and an eye mask.
- Limit the time spent in front of screens and blue light (or try the lenses that block the blue light).
- Go to bed, and I will wake up at the same time every day.

- Stop consuming coffee at noon and limit the consumption of caffeine in all its forms.
- Avoid drinking alcohol before bedtime.
- Expose yourself to natural daylight daily.

8. Reduce stress

Try stress-reduction techniques: examine the sources of stress in your life and consider if you can do something to mitigate them. Stress increases cortisol release. But don't stress by stress: it would be a dead end. During menopause, many women are in a sandwich class between still having dependent children and, at the same time, having elderly or sick parents. Loss caused by the death of loved ones is a frequent issue during the menopausal years.

When people have difficulties and face a stalemate, or have a true relapse, the number one cause is a crisis in some way in their lives. Everyone — men and women — are affected by crises. We spend a lifetime handling chaos. We recommend that people plan mechanisms to deal with stress.

Stress can also cause eating as an emotional escape, which is another cause of stagnation in weight loss or weight accumulation. Try yoga, meditation, and conscious attention, taking relaxing walks or doing other pleasant activities. A week of eating slowly and consciously where you really pay attention to flavors, textures and hunger signals. Eat slowly, deliberately and consciously.

Even worrying about your weight can cause stress. Although it may be helpful to track weight and food intake, if it becomes too stressful, the researcher recommends not doing so for a while and simply focusing on how you feel.

9. Be realistic

Some women aspire to an arbitrary figure on the scale... a figure that has nothing to do with their current health and weight.

Set realistic expectations: this advice is particularly important for women of all ages. Some women aspire to an arbitrary figure on the scale that comes from how much they weighed a long time ago or perhaps an idealized weight they never achieved, a figure that has nothing to do with your current health and weight.

It is one of the big problems I see in women, it is very entangled with psychology, self-esteem, and social pressure, and many times it is totally beyond the control of the woman in question. They get carried away by how they think they should be instead of what is really healthy for them. If you equate success with the figure on the scale, you are going to harm yourself.

Measure your success by losing centimeters and not by the figure on the scale. He advises you to accept that weight loss in middle age will be slower than when you were younger. "Remember that you are committing to this in the long term. It is an investment in health as you age. Be patient. Your long-term goal is to make a permanent change in lifestyle in addition to losing excess fat.

CHAPTER 5

WEIGHT LOSS GOAL.

When a diet has a predominance of carbohydrates, the body uses them as the main source of energy instead of fat. On the contrary, the absence of carbohydrates in the diet accelerates the use of fat. This is because insulin blocks lipolysis (by blocking the adipocyte lipase) and allows glucose to enter the fat cell. This glucose is converted into triglycerides within the adipocyte, through its transformation into acetyl-CoA and alpha-glycerophosphate (Acetyl-CoA molecules combine with each other to form fatty acids and two molecules of these fatty acids bind to one of glycerol through diacylglycerol transferase (DAGT) to form the triglyceride molecule). In addition, fatty acids from dietary fat, they need the action of glucose and insulin to be transformed into triglycerides into the fat cell, since insulin allows the entry of glucose into the adipocyte and glucose is necessary for the formation of alpha glycerophosphate, which is the main supply of glycerol to fatty acids so that they can be transformed into triglycerides and thus be stored. The last step in the synthesis of triglycerides is, therefore, the binding of glycerol to fatty acids, a reaction that is catalyzed by diacylglycerol transferase (DAGT). If for some reason, this last step does not occur, either due to a deficiency of glucose and insulin that ensures the supply of glycerol or due to a failure in the DAGT itself, it would be logical to assume that there will be an interruption in the synthesis of triglycerides. This has been demonstrated in mice with a homozygous DAGT deficiency, which was characterized by having lower white fatty tissue and being resistant to the development of dietary obesity. Therefore, low insulin levels in a ketogenic diet should produce similar effects, which would be one of the possible explanations, as we will see later, of the greater success of these diets in weight loss. It is also important to consider that glucose is not the only substance that induces the release of insulin since this process is also stimulated by certain amino acids such as arginine and lysine; Gastrointestinal hormones that are produced during intakes such as gastrin, secretin, cholecystokinin (CCK) and gastric inhibitory polypeptide (PIG). Further,

Satiating-anorexigenic effect of ketogenic diets Another important aspect to consider is the satiating effect of ketogenic diets because fats and proteins remain in the stomach for a longer period of time and are therefore able to prolong the feeling of satiety when compared to carbohydrates. In addition, cholecystokinin is considered as one of the most potent appetite suppressants and this hormone is stimulated by the consumption of fats and proteins but not by carbohydrates. This satiating effect also involves beta-hydroxybutyrate, which is the most abundant ketone and has the capacity to inhibit the appetite center directly. Also, the low glycemic index of ketogenic diets reduces fluctuations in plasma glucose concentrations; they are much more frequent with high carb diets. Thus, avoiding episodes of hypoglycemia will also reduce appetite. Another factor that must be added is that proteins have an anorexigenic effect superior to that of carbohydrates, which could be mediated by an increase in the sensitivity of the central nervous system towards leptin and a decrease in postprandial plasma concentrations of ghrelin. Leptin is produced by adipose tissue and has the ability to reduce appetite at the level of the central nervous system. However, obese people usually have circulating levels of leptin higher than normal, because there is resistance to the action of it, which would be something similar to what happens with insulin. In relation to ghrelin,

Carbohydrates could contribute to obesity

Taking into account all these physiological concepts, it would be logical to launch the hypothesis that carbohydrates alone and in large quantities can favor obesity, so that a conventional diet based on carbohydrates (50-70% of the total daily energy contribution) that exceeding a person's daily caloric needs could be more easily induced to induce obesity than a low carb diet; when consumed together with proteins, carbohydrates have the ability to multiply their obesity inducing effect; when consumed with fat, carbohydrates allow the accumulation of fat; and finally, carbohydrates have a lower satiating effect than lipids and proteins. Thus,

The activation of lipolytic metabolism triggers the appearance of ketone bodies in the blood, which is a natural response to fasting, prolonged exercise, and high-fat diets. For this reason, from a physiological point of view, weight loss strategies that are based on reducing fat intake and maintaining the proportion of carbohydrates as the main source of energy, maybe less effective for weight loss. and they would only act through a simple caloric restriction and not by a metabolic change (from glycolytic to lipolytic).

Optimal levels of carbohydrates in the ketogenic diet

The metabolic change is achieved when the carbohydrate content of the diet is low enough to cause ketosis (hence the name of ketogenic diets or too low in carbohydrates). As for the level of carbohydrates that a diet must have to be considered ketogenic, it is necessary to make actualizations, since this will depend on the end of said diet. If a ketogenic diet is used to lose weight, the amount of carbohydrates ingested should be less than 0.2-0.4g / kg of weight and day, being able to consume fat and protein without any restriction. On the contrary, when the ketogenic diet is used for the treatment of epilepsy in children, this diet must be much more restrictive in order to achieve much stronger ketosis, such that the carbohydrate content must be very low: less than 10 g per day. In addition, this ketogenic diet is also low in protein and very high in fat so that the fat-non-fat ratio (protein + carbohydrates) is of the order of 4: 1 (9-12).

At equal calories, the ketogenic diet is more efficient in weight loss

The fact that at the same number of calories, the ketogenic diet is more effective than a low-fat diet, can only be explained by its lower metabolic efficiency. This is due to the fact that, from a physiological point of view, there is an association between plasma levels and urinary ketone levels, in addition to the fact that acetone is characterized by being volatile and therefore partly eliminated through the breath. This would mean an energy loss through urinary elimination and breath of ketones. In addition, if we consider that ketogenic diets do not produce hypoglycemia, but quite the opposite, since they improve the glycemic profile, we should assume that gluconeogenesis plays a prominent role. In this gluconeogenic process, there is also a significant energy loss, due to the fact that 100 g of medium quality protein are needed to form only 57 g of glucose, which would mean an energy loss of approximately 43% if we assume the energy equivalence that 1 g of glucose provides approximately the same energy as 1 g of protein, i.e., 4-5 Kcal / g. In fact, it has been proven that the endogenous breakdown of 110 g of protein, which is necessary to form approximately 60 to 65 g of glucose, supposes a daily energy loss of approximately 400-600 kcal / day. In addition, during the formation of one mole of glucose from the alanine, six moles of ATP are lost. This energy loss is very significant since one mole of glucose gives 38 ATP so that the loss of six moles of ATP would mean an energy loss of almost 16% in the gluconeogenic process from the alanine, which is metabolically easier than for other amino acids because they have chemical configurations that hinder this process. For this reason, an energy loss of 43% should not surprise us.

This lower metabolic efficiency and the anorexigenic effect of the proteins could justify that the protein intake is inversely associated with abdominal obesity in multiethnic populations, probably this influences the genetic predisposition to develop insulin resistance, which as we know is associated with the Central obesity already diets high in carbohydrates while improving with protein-rich diets. Together with the lower metabolic efficiency, we must emphasize that insulin is necessary for the formation of triglycerides and that high-fat diets increase energy loss through the activation of thermogenesis since it has been proven that the expression of decoupling proteins or thermogenins (PCU), responsible for the thermogenesis process,

All these arguments would explain why at equal calorie ketogenic diets are more effective than carbohydrate-rich diets in weight loss.

Studies that corroborate the effectiveness of ketogenic diets in weight loss

At the same number of calories, ketogenic diets are more effective in weight loss than conventional high-carb and low-fat diets, in addition to having the added advantage of being more selective in fat loss and mass muscle preservation (13,28). Benoit et al. showed that when a ketogenic diet of 1000 kcal per day (10 g of carbohydrates per day) was followed for 10 days, the subjects involved lost an average of 600 g of weight per day, of which 97% was fat. Young et al. compared three diets with the same amount of calories (1800 kcal / day) but with a different proportion of carbohydrates (104 g, 60 g and 30 g respectively) and observed a negative correlation between the proportion of carbohydrates in the diet and weight loss and a positive correlation with the loss of lean mass. So that the lower-carb diet was better when it came to losing weight and preserving muscle mass. Willi et al. also found in their study that the use of a low carb diet in morbidly obese adolescents was an effective method for weight loss and mass muscle preservation. Also, in another study with adolescents, Sondike et al. found that a low carb diet without caloric restriction in fat and protein was more effective in weight loss and improved blood lipid profile than using a low-fat diet.

These authors went further in their statements stating that in adolescents who had followed a low carb diet without calorie restriction in fat and protein, despite consuming an average of more than 700 Kcal daily than the group that followed a low-fat diet, the weight loss was more than double and the improvement in the most pronounced triglyceride level. These statements are also shared by Greene et al. , which showed that at the same number of Kcal, and even increasing their number by 300 or more, low carbohydrate diets achieved greater weight loss than low-fat diets. Samaha et al. conducted a six-month study in which they found that people with morbid obesity and a high prevalence of type II diabetes or metabolic syndrome, lost a greater weight during this period of time in the low carb diet that The diet low in calories and fat, with an improvement in insulin sensitivity and triglyceride levels, even after adjusting to the amount of weight loss that as we know is a factor that can influence the results.

On the other hand, Yancy et al. concluded in another six-month study that the low-carb diet had a higher percentage of adherence and weight loss success compared to a low-fat diet. they lost more weight during this period of time in the low carb diet than the low calorie and fat diet, with improved insulin sensitivity and triglyceride levels, even after adjusting to the amount of weight loss that, as we know, is a factor that can influence the results. On the other hand, Yancy et al. concluded in another six-month study that the low-carb diet had a higher percentage of adherence and weight loss success compared to a low-fat diet. they lost more weight during this period of time in the low carb diet than the low calorie and fat diet, with improved insulin sensitivity and triglyceride levels, even after adjusting the amount of weight loss that, as we know, is a factor that can influence the results. On the other hand, Yancy et al. concluded in another six-month study that the low-carb diet had a higher percentage of adherence and weight loss success compared to a low-fat diet. Even after adjusting the amount of weight loss that as we know, it is a factor that can influence the results. On the other hand, Yancy et al. concluded in another six-month study that the low-carb diet had a higher percentage of adherence and weight loss success compared to a low-fat diet. Even after adjusting the amount of weight loss that as we know, it is a factor that can influence the results. On the other hand, Yancy et al. concluded in another six-month study that the low-carb diet had a higher percentage of adherence and weight loss success compared to a low-fat diet.

Long term studies

The main limitation attributed to studies for weight loss performed with ketogenic diets is that they are studies that never exceed two years. However, we should also take into account that there are also no rigorous studies in the scientific literature, with conventional hypocaloric diets continuously that exceed that period. This could have a logical explanation, and generally, there are usually no patients who are willing to follow any type of diet uninterruptedly for a period of time that goes beyond 1-2 years. Therefore, serious studies cannot be done with a certain number of patients who undertake to follow this diet for such a long period of time. This is probably due, Because generally in this period of time, they usually lose the desired weight or lose the motivation necessary to continue with the same diet. For this reason, the strategy followed by many nutritionists is to reach a certain weight with a more aggressive diet focused on weight loss, maintain that weight for a certain time with a less restrictive and more enjoyable maintenance diet, and if the patient needs to lose more weight, re-enter the diet used at the beginning.

As we saw earlier, in studies of up to six months duration, ketogenic diets are more effective than conventional high-calorie low-carb diets for weight loss, however, as we will see later, when the duration increases, the effectiveness of these diets is reduced and equals that of conventional hypocaloric diets. What we will never know is whether this is due to the nature of the diet itself or to the strict breach of it by the patient, which could increase as the duration of the diet increases. Foster et al. and Stern et al. compared ketogenic low carb diets versus traditional diets (low calorie-fat and carbohydrate-rich diets) for weight loss for one year.

In both clinical trials, the low carb diet produced greater weight loss than conventional diets during the first six months, although the differences were not significant at a one-year duration. In both diets, the authors stated that adherence was poor. However, the participants in the group of low carbohydrate diets had overall more favorable results per year than conventional diets, since they showed a greater improvement in some factors of cardiovascular risk (higher levels of HDL and lower triglyceride levels) and in the improvement of glycemic control after having adjusted the differences to weight loss. In another study, in which Dansinger et al. compared four types of diets (ketogenic, from the area, of the points and Ornish) observed that after one year of duration, adherence was generally poor for the four types of diet, although people who had greater adherence to any of the groups also had a greater improvement in weight loss and in cardiovascular risk factors. Brinkworth et al., in a clinical trial in which they compared two groups, one treated with a standard protein diet and another with a high protein diet, stated that in the 17th month of follow-up, adherence was poor in both groups. Finally, in another 14-month study conducted with obese diabetic patients, Dasthi et al. They observed that people who followed the ketogenic diet had a progressive improvement not only in weight but also in glucose levels, total cholesterol,

Taking into account all these studies, the real problem associated with long-term diets, whether ketogenic or not, is low adherence because people end up getting bored with the same eating patterns so that to achieve high Adhesion, these people need a great personal effort. Considering that people with morbid obesity usually have associated cardiovascular problems and that in industrialized countries there are many overweight people who do not reach the degree of obesity bitten, so they will only need to lose weight for a short period of time, low diets in carbohydrates they could be of choice in both cases thanks to the substantial advantages they present compared to conventional high-carb diets.

In people with low weight, low carb diets would also be useful because they will improve body composition: they will reduce fat and increase muscle mass. The conservation of muscle mass associated with this type of diet seems to be related to ketones since it has been proven that they have the ability to reduce protein catabolism in catabolic situations such as fasting.

Another undoubted advantage presented by ketogenic diets over traditional hypocaloric diets in patients who follow them is the feeling of satiety and loss of hunger they cause, improvement in mood, energy levels, mental and physical state, while traditional low-calorie carbohydrate-rich diets can even increase appetite and are associated with a worsening in both mental and physical state.

Are they safe in the long term?

Contrary to the general opinion, the ketogenic diets used for weight loss are effective and safe for long periods of time. Thus Westman et al. stated that obese women who followed a pure ketogenic diet without caloric restriction in fat and protein (carbohydrates <25 g / day) maintained weight loss and improved lipid profile — for periods of one year, comparing a pure ketogenic diet without caloric restriction in fats and proteins (carbohydrates <30 g daily) with a conventional low-calorie low-calorie-high-carbohydrate diet (<30% daily fat energy), The ketogenic diet was found to be healthier since it was associated with a greater improvement in cardiovascular risk factors and in the glycemic index.

Despite these studies, there are scientists who continue to distrust these types of diets because they argue that there are no studies of more than two years, so that monitoring these types of diets for a lifetime could have very negative consequences on the health of the person. Faced with this opinion, it is worth mentioning that, in the evolution of the human diet, the human being had followed a hunter-gatherer diet in which the carbohydrates throughout most of their evolution (approximately 2 million years) they were consumed in very low quantities and only when the time of the year allowed it. While the transition to a diet based on carbohydrates, What is currently considered the ideal food? It has a very short duration in the evolutionary period of our species (approximately 6000 years ago, with the introduction of agriculture and livestock). This dietary change was associated with obesity, cardiovascular problems and dental losses, as evidenced by the archeological findings found in the mummies of ancient Egypt, a civilization in which the negative consequences of such change could be seen very significantly. Without going any further, many current tribes who followed ketogenic diets and who have adopted the dietary system based on carbohydrates, such as the Eskimos (diet based on fish and marine mammals such as the seal), they have experienced a worsening in atherogenic plasma markers and in the development of diseases that were previously virtually unknown in these populations, such as type II diabetes and central obesity. It could also influence this worsening of health, the lower content of polyunsaturated fatty acids that this population experienced as a result of said dietary change.

CHAPTER 6

IMPLEMENTATION OF PHYSICAL ACTIVITY

Exercises for the elderly - Starting to do fitness at age 50. Making a little history, for a long time, the 50-year-old woman was thought of as someone older, someone who already had her life done. Reality has changed and today a 50-year-old person is fully active, worries about keeping his body moving and attends to the different alternatives offered by the market for it.

We all know or have heard, on occasion the benefits of physical activity, but what does this concept contain? It is directly associated with health. It is true that there are many people who start a gym because it was recommended by the doctor, but there are also other people who go because they want to feel good. It's like that! Today a woman of 50 years or more is not only fully active but also goes for more. Looking for exercise, but also looking for fun.

In this sense, in the world of fitness, there is a diversity of exercises for older women to choose from. Now, let's focus on what is recommended. From my experience, I can say that when a person starts a physical activity, whatever it is, it has to be pleasant. Otherwise, leave. That on the one hand.

On the other, regarding the physical activity that this group can develop (people 50 years and older), it is very varied. Beyond assuming that the more years a person is in, the less physical activity they must do, it is totally false. As time goes by, we have to think that, obviously, just as muscle tissue decreases, we can also sustain that tone and without too much sacrifice. Enough 30 minutes a day of exercise for older people with some weights, not large, to recover that lost muscle tissue in a period not so long.

Breaking with beliefs

When a student enters the gym for the first time with more than 50 years, he thinks that he is in a very bad physical condition to work with weights, or that training with weights implies having a lot of muscle, or that it is a training for people younger. What he does not think, or does not know is that exercising with weights is the best way to get in shape and recover the tone of the muscles.

If we don't work the muscles, every year, we lose an average of 500g of muscle tissue. There, our worst enemies of old age begin to emerge: physical ailments in general, loss of strength, resistance, metabolism reduction, etc. However, it has been shown that older people who train with weights three times a week significantly increase their mineral bone content.

Most people find it hard to find the time, but above all, they want to exercise. And yet, if you accustom the body to being in motion, when you skip your exercise routine, it starts to hurt everything.

A well-exercised body stays more elastic, healthier, and more energetic for more years. It is, in large part, what has made some people reach the fifties in a relatively good way. Of course, it is never too late to start.

Most people find it hard to find the time, but above all, they want to exercise. And yet, if you accustom the body to being in motion, when you skip your exercise routine, it starts to hurt everything from the back to the legs. That should be enough motivation to put on your shoes and run for a few kilometers.

Although some are runners from a young age, they do not recommend this sport for people who start a sporting routine in middle age, because running has its disadvantages - it is not the best for the knees or the back. Of course, it is great to combat stress. Let's see what are the best routines from the age of fifty and why based on the experience and knowledge of some physical trainers.

The best Exercise for a woman over 50 to weight loss

Walking: It has many advantages. It is free (unless you do it on the gym treadmill), it is low impact, it can be done anywhere and does not require great physical preparation. Taking your dog or your grandson for a walk in his baby carriage is one of the best excuses to go for a walk. Half an hour a day is better than nothing, but if you can do it for an hour every day, even better.

Swimming: It has always been considered one of the best exercises for older people. It is one of the complete sports because, in addition to providing cardiovascular benefits, it requires that you move all major muscle groups. One of the biggest advantages it has is that the risk of injuring yourself by swimming is minimal by the means in which you do it - water. It has the disadvantage that you have to go to a pool, wet your hair, protect your eyes, so I reserve it for the summer.

Dancing: It's another of my favorite activities. Be it salsa, ballroom dancing, jazz, Zumba; it also has many advantages. On the one hand, it forces you to leave home and sometimes even dress and get ready for the occasion. On the other hand, when you dance, you have to think about the next step you are going to take, and it is a great coordination exercise. This is very important as we turn years because it keeps agile not only the body but also the mind and emotions. And finally, when you dance, you can't think of anything else. It is a form of meditation.

Yoga: The benefits of yoga include increased flexibility, muscle toning, and emotional therapy. People seem to believe that over the years, losing elasticity is inevitable. No, it is not. At 51, you can still touch your feet without bending your knees; in fact, there are older people who have an enviable elasticity. In addition, yoga helps control the emotional ups and downs that the onset of the menopause era entails.

Resistance exercises: Since the forties, but especially after menopause (in the case of women), they lose muscle mass and gain fat. In addition, the risk of osteoporosis increases. All this is due to the hormonal changes in these stages. Fortunately, this can be counteracted with resistance exercises. You can use your own bodyweight to do push-ups or lift weights. And remember, with each birthday, it becomes even more important to make an effort to exercise the body. The weights will not only help you to have beautiful arms but also a strong body and more resistant to falls and disease.

Of course, before starting any exercise routine, especially if you are not used to sports, consult your doctor. Also, remember that you don't need to prepare for a triathlon, but why not? There is the case of several women who have rediscovered themselves in middle age, thanks to sports.

The best Exercise for a woman over 50 for a Longevity life

Iron: Strengthens arms, chest, abdomen, hips, and legs. Start with an iron-on your knees, and over time you can make the whole iron.

- **Execution:** Put the entire body straight, like a board, with the feet and the tips of the feet on the mat and the hands directly under your chest. Using your arms, go down to the count of 4 and return to the count of 4. Do 12-15 repetitions.

Squat: Work the lower body, thighs, hips, and buttocks.

- **Execution:** Stand with your feet under your hips, shoulder width. Extend your arms in front of you to keep your balance (or lean on the back of a chair).

Slowly bend your knees, with your chest and buttocks out, and stop once you are almost "sitting in a chair." It is essential that you remove your buttocks as much as possible as you go down to maintain pressure on your knees. Do 15 repetitions.

Squat: It focuses on the thighs, a problem area for many women.

- **Execution:** Stand with your feet wider than your hip. Turn your feet out and your heels in. Slowly bring your weight back from the body on your heels as you bend your knees to your toes and squat with your buttocks out. Never put the tailbone, because this puts a lot of pressure on the knees.

Table: It is a hard exercise, but the whole body works.

- **Execution:** Keep your body in a plank position, staying perfectly still for 30-60 seconds. Keep your abs contracted and your back straight all the time, try to reach 60 seconds.

Abdominals: They help maintain good posture and relieve back pressure as you get older.

- **Execution:** lie down with your back completely flat, with your hands behind your head, tuck your belly button towards the floor and use your abdominal muscles to go up and then down. Exhale as it rises and inhale when it falls. Keep your legs and feet flat on the floor and see if you can do 20 in 60 seconds.

CHAPTER 7

WHAT TO EAT TO LOSE WEIGHT WITH THE KETONIC DIET?

The ketogenic diet is to be reasonable in your food choices. It's up to you to make personal choices in some areas of the keto diet. But like most things in life, if you consume certain foods, do it in moderation. Portion sizes are also important, as, in most diet plans, you must make sure that you do not eat half a cow in one meal, for example.

Do not spend or waste your time making yourself feel guilty if you eat something that is not included in the ketogenic diet. You should congratulate yourself for trying to make positive changes in your life by trying to change your eating habits. Let's face it; changing bad habits will require work and discipline. But the keto diet recipes in this book will give you the impression that you appreciate this new way of eating healthier, it will not seem like a punishment, and it will not only please your taste buds, but it will also improve your health!

To start a ketogenic diet, you should be more restrictive about your carbohydrate intake (less than 15g per day), which will allow you to enter ketosis faster and improve your overall results. Most of your meals should consist of protein, vegetables, and a fat supplement.

The ketogenic diet does not simply limit the consumption of carbohydrates but urges us to reduce their use to a quantity with which we can live. Of course, those who exercise regularly can afford to eat more carbs than the rest of us, but the idea is to eat only the carbohydrates that your body will use immediately.

Carbohydrates should come mainly from vegetables, nuts, dark green leafy vegetables, and dairy products. It is also crucial to avoid refined carbohydrates (such as wheat products), starch (such as potatoes and legumes) or fruits.

Eat all types of meat (poultry, beef, pork, and fish) and all kinds of fat. However, olive oil and coconut are much better.

If you are hungry and craving carbs throughout the day, you can nibble nuts, peanut butter, seeds, or cheese to appease your appetite.

Dairy products:

- Heavy whipped cream
- Cheese
- Greek yogurt
- Mayonnaise (preferably homemade)
- Mascarpone, fresh cream
- Soft cheese, including mozzarella, brie, blue, etc.
- Hard cheese such as aged cheddar, parmesan cheese, feta cheese, and Swiss cheese

Seeds and nuts:

- Nuts
- Almonds
- Cashew nut
- Pistachio
- Flour of seeds
- Sunflower seeds
- Chia seeds

Drinks:

- Broth
- Almond milk
- Water
- Coffee

- Coconut milk
- Herbal teas

Fats and oils:

- Animal fat (non-hydrogenated)
- Lard
- lawyers
- Egg yolks
- Macadamia / Brazil nuts
- Butter / Ghee
- Coconut butter
- Cocoa butter
- Olive oil
- Coconut oil
- Avocado oil
- Macadamia oil

Fruits:

- Strawberries
- Blueberries
- Raspberries
- Cherries
- Cranberries
- Blackberry

Vegetables:

- Kale
- Spinach
- Chard
- Salad
- Radi
- Brussels sprouts
- Broccoli

Other options:

- Onions
- Peppers
- Asparagus
- Celery
- Cucumber
- Squash
- Cauliflower

Protein:

- Fish
- Red meat
- Poultry
- Pork
- Whole eggs
- Bacon
- Seafood

- Peanut Butter
- Lamb
- Goat

Spices:

- Cayenne pepper
- Chili powder
- Cinnamon
- Cumin
- Oregano
- Basil
- Parsley
- Rosemary
- Thyme

Condiments and sauces:

- Ketchup
- Mustard
- Mayonnaise
- Worcestershire sauce
- Ranch vinaigrette
- Flavored syrups (with acceptable sweeteners)

Sweeteners:

- Stevia

- Sucralose
- Erythritol
- Monk fruit

We should carefully choose vegetables on a ketogenic diet since they play an important role in any healthy meal. Some of them are loaded with sugar, so choose vegetables rich in nutrients and fiber. You can use green leaves and eat them whenever you want to increase your fiber intake.

Also, scan the product labels and check their carbohydrate content before purchase.

CHAPTER 8

AN EXCELLENT KETO MEAL PLAN FOR A WEEK

A ketogenic healthy diet should revolve around high fat, low carb food choices, and limit highly processed items and unhealthy fats. Keto-friendly drink choices must be sugar-free. Think about water, sparkling water, or green tea without sugar and coffee.

The following menu provides less than 50 grams of carbohydrates a day in total.

As mentioned above, some people may have to reduce carbohydrates even more to achieve ketosis.

This one-week general ketogenic menu can be modified according to dietary needs.

On Monday

- **Breakfast** - Breakfast: two fried eggs in served butter with greens sauteed grazed.
- **Lunch:** A bunless grass-fed hamburger garnished with cheese, mushrooms, and avocado on a bed of green vegetables.

- **Dinner:** Pork chops with green beans sautéed in coconut oil.

Tuesday

- **Breakfast** - Breakfast: a mushroom omelet.
- **Lunch:** Tuna salad with celery and tomato on a bed of green vegetables.
- **Dinner:** Roasted chicken with cream sauce and broccoli sauteed.

Wednesday

- **Breakfast** - Breakfast: Peppers stuffed with cheese and eggs.
- **Lunch:** Arugula salad with boiled eggs, turkey, avocado, and blue cheese.
- **Dinner:** grilled salmon with spinach sautéed in coconut oil.

Thursday

- **Breakfast** - Breakfast: fat yogurt topped with granola full Keto.
- **Lunch:** Steak bowl with cauliflower rice, cheese, herbs, avocado, and salsa.
- **Dinner:** Bison steak with cheesy broccoli.

Friday

- **Breakfast -** Lunch: Avocado Egg boat oven.
- **Lunch:** Caesar salad with chicken.
- **Dinner:** Pork chops with vegetables.

Saturday

- **Breakfast -** Breakfast: toast Chou - flower topped with cheese and avocado.
- **Lunch:** Salmon burgers with bunless pesto topped.
- **Dinner:** meatballs served with zucchini noodles and parmesan cheese.

Sunday

- **Breakfast -** Breakfast: of Milk coconut chia pudding garnished with nuts coconut and nuts.
- **Lunch:** Cobb salad with vegetables, boiled eggs, avocado, cheese, and turkey.
- **Dinner:** chicken with coconut curry.

As you can see, ketogenic meals can be diverse and tasty.

Although many ketogenic meals are based on animal products, there is a wide variety of vegetarian options to choose from as well.

If you follow a more liberal ketogenic diet, adding a cup of berries to your breakfast or a small portion of a starchy food at your dinner will increase the carbohydrate count in this meal plan.

Summary

A ketogenic meal plan, like any healthy diet, should include whole foods and many, low-carb, high fiber vegetables. Choose healthy fats such as coconut oil, avocado, olive oil, and butter to increase the fat content of the dishes.

Ketogenic Healthy Snack Options

Between meals can snacking help moderate hunger and keep you on track by following a ketogenic diet.

Because the ketogenic diet is so filling, you may only need one or two snacks a day, depending on your activity level.

Here are some excellent, ketonic-friendly snacks:

- Almonds and cheddar cheese
- Half avocado stuffed with chicken salad
- Guacamole with low carb vegetables
- Trail mix made with unsweetened coconut, nuts, and seeds

- Hard-boiled eggs
- coconut chips
- Kale chips
- Olives and sliced salami
- Celery and peppers with cream cheese dip with herbs
- Berries with whipping cream
- Jerky
- Cheese roll-ups
- parmesan chips
- Macadamia nuts
- Greens with creamy fat dressing and avocado
- Keto Smoothie made with coconut milk, cocoa, and avocado
- Avocado cocoa mousse

Although these ketone snacks can maintain fullness between meals, they can also contribute to weight gain if you are snacking too much throughout the day.

It is important to eat the appropriate number of calories based on your activity level, the goal of weight loss, age, and sex.

Summary

Keto-friendly snacks should be high in fat, moderate in protein, and low in carbohydrates. Increase your fiber intake by nibbling on slices, low-carb veggies with a high- fat sauce.

A Simple Commercial Ketogenic List

A well-rounded ketogenic diet should include lots of fresh products, healthy fats, and proteins. Choosing a mix of both fresh and frozen products will ensure that you have an offer of vegetables and keto-friendly fruits to add to the recipes.

What follows is a simple ketogenic shopping list that can guide you when browsing the grocery aisles:

- **Meat and poultry:** beef, chicken, turkey, and pork (choose organic products and raised in the pasture where possible).
- **Fish:** Fatty fish such as salmon, sardines, mackerel, and herring arc the best.
- **Seafood:** oysters, shrimps, and scallops.
- **Eggs:** Purchase enriched omega-3 or eggs whenever possible.
- **Dairy products high in fat:** unsweetened yogurt, butter, cream, and sour cream.
- **Oils:** Coconut coconut and avocado oil.

- **Avocados:** Buy a mixture of blackberries and unripe avocados so that your diet will last.
- **Cheese:** Brie, cream cheese, cheddar cheese, and goat cheese.
- **Frozen or fresh berries:** Blueberries, raspberries, blackberries.
- **Nuts:** Nuts macadamia, almonds, walnuts pecans, pistachios.
- **Seeds:** The seeds of pumpkin, sunflower seeds, seeds chia.
- **Nut butter:** almond butter, peanut butter.
- **Fresh or frozen low carbohydrate vegetables:** mushrooms, cauliflower, broccoli, greens, peppers, onions, and tomatoes.
- **Condiments:** sea salt, pepper, salsa, herbs, garlic, vinegar, mustard, olives, and spices.

It is always helpful to plan your meals and fill your basket with the necessary ingredients to a few days' worths of healthy dishes. Plus, sticking to a shopping list can help you avoid unhealthy, tempting foods.

Summary

Preparing a shopping list can help you decide which foods will fit into your ketogenic meal plan.

Fill your basket with meat, poultry, eggs, low carb vegetables, whole milk, and healthy fats.

The Bottom Line

A healthy ketogenic diet should consist of approximately 75% fat, 20% protein, and only 5% or less than 50 grams of carbohydrate a day.

Focus on high fat, low carbohydrate foods such as eggs, meats, dairy, and low carb vegetables, as well as sugar-free beverages. Be sure to limit highly processed items and unhealthy fats.

Using this book as a guide to starting on the keto diet plan can put you in place to succeed and make the transition to a high-fat, low-carb diet a breeze.

CHAPTER 9

FOOD TO COMPLETELY AVOID

The review of different food families has shown us that in the ketogenic diet, it is important to eliminate or reduce the consumption of carbohydrates. They prevent the passage from the state of ketosis. As you can see, carbohydrates are almost everywhere ... even in simple lettuce. Hence the importance of being attentive to each food consumed and of making calculations to restore balance, at least at the start of your "ketogenic" adventure in order to take your bearings and adapt your habits. More generally, be aware that there are too many carbohydrates in the food families detailed in this chapter, and that their consumption should be restricted as much as possible, or even eliminated.

No to cereals

Particularly rich in carbohydrates, cereals must be limited in the diet when they are raw and complete (such as whole rice, quinoa, oatmeal, corn kernels...) eliminated completely when they are refined or processed (flour, dough, bread, cookies, breakfast cereals...). Do you miss all these products? Be aware that there are tips to replace them.

Instead of bread. Some crunchy sandwiches rich in fiber (based on various seeds, a little flour...) can help you out. Check their carbohydrate content carefully: some display around 4 g of carbohydrates per slice, which is quite reasonable. High protein bread (in supermarkets, some bakers) can also be a good option, but check their composition because not all are equal. There are also several ways to make ketogenic "bread" or seed crackers that can replace traditional bread.

Instead of flour. In cakes, pancakes, or pie crusts, you can use almond powder and / or coconut flour. Powdered cauliflower can also be used as "flour," especially in making pizza dough.

In place of the potato. For a delicious homemade puree, try the cauliflower, which is an excellent substitute. To thicken a vegetable soup, the zucchini performs the same role as a binder as the potato.

Instead of pasta. Zucchini spaghetti is an illusion. Also, try products made from konjac (like shirataki), a plant rich in fiber and very low in carbohydrates and calories. This star food in Japan satisfies for the long term and is considered a real slimming remedy. Only drawback: its tasteless taste and its texture which can confuse!

Instead of rice. Test the cauliflower rice! It can also perfectly replace semolina for a "tabbouleh." There is also khanjac Gohan (or rice).

Note, however, whole rice and organic (unrefined) oats can be kept as part of a low carb diet.

Long Live Ketogenic Food!

Beware of industrial dishes

They have no place in the ketogenic diet, and this for several reasons:

- Most are rich in various and varied additives, and in particular, in added sugars that play the role of preservatives or enhancers of taste.
- The quality of the fats used is often poor, generally for economic reasons. Most of the time, they are hydrogenated fats (even if in recent years, manufacturers have made efforts to reduce them) or too rich in omega-6.

Conclusion: always check the nutritional composition of the industrial dishes you buy, as well as their carbohydrate content

Some can help out but prefer homemade lunch boxes or dishes cooked by chefs, delivered to your home, or your workplace if you can.

Little note to galvanize you: it still depends on the goal to be achieved and the reason for this ketogenic diet. It should be remembered that paleo can be an "easy made" alternative for motivated but somewhat cautious people to a strict ketogenic, or quite simply for a person refractory to cooking and precise calculations. Let's stay cool!

Sugar and sugary foods: limit as much as possible

Is it worth pointing out that sugar and very sweet products (jam, candy, ice cream...) have no place in the ketogenic diet? For sweet beaks, we will always prefer "intelligent" sugars, rich in minerals (honey, maple syrup, agave syrup). They are, however, to be avoided if one wishes to follow a strict ketogenic diet.

As for sugar itself, the ketogenic diet will gradually get you used to its taste, and you will soon be able to do without it. Still, at the start of the diet, sweeteners can be useful for you not to crack. But beware, not just any.

Stevia: it is certainly the best option. Extracted from a plant, this 100% natural sweetener contains neither calories nor carbohydrates. It can also be used in baking. Its sweetening power is very high (200 to 300 times more than that of sugar) pay attention to the dosage. In general, a very small pinch is enough to sweeten a coffee or tea for example. The only drawback: an aftertaste of licorice which some people may not like. It is found in raw form (it is green in color) or refined (in white color), in powder or in the liquid version. Check the label of the product you choose: many manufacturers combine stevia with other types of sweeteners. Real stevia only contains stevia.

Not all other sweeteners are created equal. A distinction must be made between artificial and therefore synthetic sweeteners (such as aspartame, saccharin, acesulfame-K, saccharin, etc.) and natural sweeteners derived from plants (such as polyols, which are alcoholic sugar, erythritol...). In addition, who says sweetener does not necessarily mean the absence of calories and the absence of carbohydrates. Some contain a little more than others. Some of the best choices include erythritol (available online), a natural sugar found in fruits, vegetables, and some fermented foods. It has no effect on blood sugar levels because it is quickly eliminated. Its sweetening power is close to that of sugar and it is well suited for baking.

Also, be aware that other natural products can play the role of sweeteners. Certain spices, such as cinnamon or vanilla, naturally soften a drink or a dairy product. Cinnamon has the virtue of stimulating insulin and therefore reducing the level of blood sugar. A real plus to favor. Do not hesitate to use them to replace sugar. Other products also allow you to naturally "sweeten" your desserts. This is the case, for example, with coconut milk, oilseed "flours" (almond powder, coconut flour...)

Sweeteners, Dangerous For Health?

The safety of sweeteners is often questioned. Know that today, scientists agree that the most important is to respect daily consumption limits: for example 40 mg per kg of body weight for aspartame (i.e., 24 g per day for a person of 60 kg), 15 mg per kg of body weight for sucralose (i.e., 9 g per day for a 60 kg person), 4 mg per kg of body weight for stevia (i.e., 2.4 g for a 60 kg person)... Knowing that a teaspoon of sweetener is 0.5 g, or that a tiny pinch of stevia is enough to sweeten a drink, there is room!

In general, also know that sweeteners, whether artificial or natural, maintain the taste of sugar. As part of a ketogenic diet, their use can be occasional, to sweeten a dessert, and this is quite appreciable. But be aware that the more you eat sweet-tasting food, the more you will want to eat it! The ketogenic diet is certainly an opportunity to get used to it.

Another essential sweet product: chocolate. Can't live without it? Note that it is not prohibited under certain conditions.

Unsweetened cocoa powder can be used as part of the ketogenic diet because its carbohydrate content remains acceptable (9 g per 100 g).

The chocolate bar is also allowed, provided you consume it in moderation, and not choose any. Opt for chocolate with 70 or 86% minimum cocoa, because it has the best carbohydrate / fat ratio. Be aware that the more chocolate is rich in cocoa, the more it is rich in fat and less in sugar. Thus, a 40% cocoa chocolate can have a carbohydrate content of more than 54 g and lipid content of 30 g. In contrast, 99% of chocolate can display around 10 g of carbohydrates for the fat content of about 50 g.

These values vary of course depending on the brand chosen: always check them on the labels.

Sweet drinks and alcohol: keep an eye out!

Sugary drinks (fruit juices, syrups, sodas...) are, of course, prohibited because they are too rich in carbohydrates.

Also, watch out for "light," "sugar-free," or "0%" drinks. The simple sweet taste stimulates the desire to consume sweet. These products include sweeteners in their composition instead of sugar, so the sweet taste remains. Be careful because if some of these sugar alternatives display 0 carbohydrates, this is not the case for all. Result: some light products (such as drinks, sodas) can be rich in carbohydrates. Always check it on the label, and don't forget to count them in your daily ratio if you consume them.

Also, be aware that some alcohols have a high carbohydrate content. Avoid beer and very sweet alcohol like port, which contain about 12 g of carbohydrates per dose. Avoid very sweet cocktails. Rather bet on red and white wines... to consume in moderation of course. Be careful, however, to take it into account in your calculations because alcohol sugar is very caloric: 7

calories per 1 gram. A glass of white or red wine or champagne provides a hundred calories per glass.

AUTHORIZED BEVERAGES

- Water. It should become your number 1 drink.

- Coffee and tea. Consume with moderation because they can have exciting effects in some people. Be aware that for others, coffee prevents ketosis, but nothing is proven. One thing is certain: do not decorate them with sugar and milk, but prefer crème fraîche, even butter and coconut oil (as in bulletproof coffee).

- Classic herbal teas and herbal teas made with fruit. Warning , these can be more or less rich in carbohydrates, check it on the label.

CHAPTER 10

BREAKFAST RECIPES

Some people skip breakfast because they think it will help them lose weight, but skipping meals is not good, because you may miss the opportunity to eat essential nutrients.

There is scientific evidence to suggest that breakfast consumption can help people control their weight as it helps activate metabolism and control appetite.

Omelet Caprese

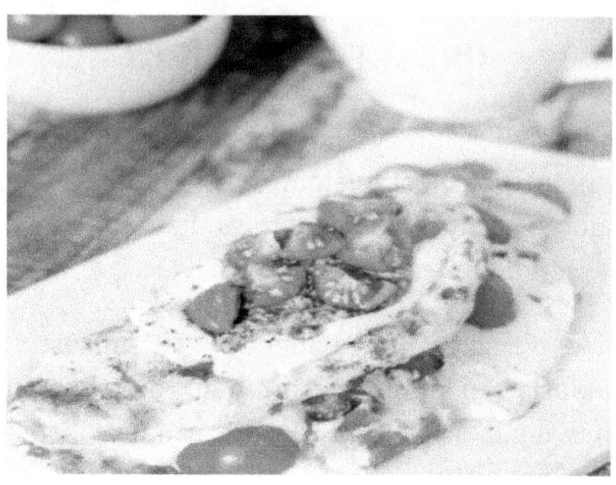

Prep time: 5 mins

2 portions

Ingredients

- 2 tbsp olive oil
- Six eggs
- 100g cherry tomatoes, cut in halves or tomatoes cut into slices
- 1 tbsp fresh basil or dried basil
- 150 g (325 ml) fresh mozzarella cheese
- salt and pepper

Preparations

1. Break the eggs in a bowl to mix and add salt and black pepper to taste. Beat well with a

fork until everything is completely mixed. Add basil and stir.

2. Cut the tomatoes into halves or slices. Chop or slice the cheese.
3. Heat the oil in a large skillet. Fry the tomatoes for a few minutes.
4. Pour the egg mixture over the tomatoes. Wait until it becomes a little firm and add the cheese.
5. Lower the heat and let the omelet harden. Serve immediately, and enjoy!

Nutrition fact

Ketogenic low in carbons

Per portion

- Net carbohydrates: 3% (4 g)
- Fiber: 1 g
- Fats: 73% (45 g)
- Protein: 24% (33 g)
- kcal: 560

Scrambled Eggs

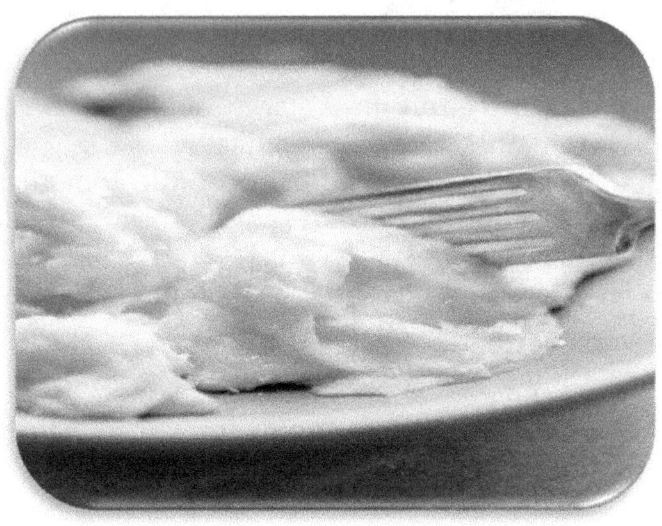

Prep time: 5 mins

1 portion

Ingredients

- Two eggs
- 30 g butter
- Salt and ground black pepper

Preparations

1. Beat the eggs together with some salt and pepper using a fork.

2. Melt the butter in a nonstick skillet over medium heat. Look closely: butter does not turn golden!
3. Pour the eggs into the pan and mix for 1-2 minutes until they are creamy and cooked a little less than you like. Remember that the eggs will continue to cook even once you put them on your plate.

Tips!

- These creamy eggs, pair well with many popular low carb dishes. Of course, there is the option of eating them with classic accompaniments such as bacon or sausage, but there are other great options such as salmon, avocado, cold cuts and cheese (cheddar, fresh mozzarella or feta).
- And if you're very hungry (or are cooking with large eggs), do not be shy: use more butter!

Nutrition fact

Ketogenic low in carbons

For portion

- Net carbohydrates: 1% (1 g)
- Fiber: 0 g
- Fat: 85% (31 g)
- Protein: 14% (11 g)
- kcal: 327

Keto Eggs With Avocado And Bacon Candles

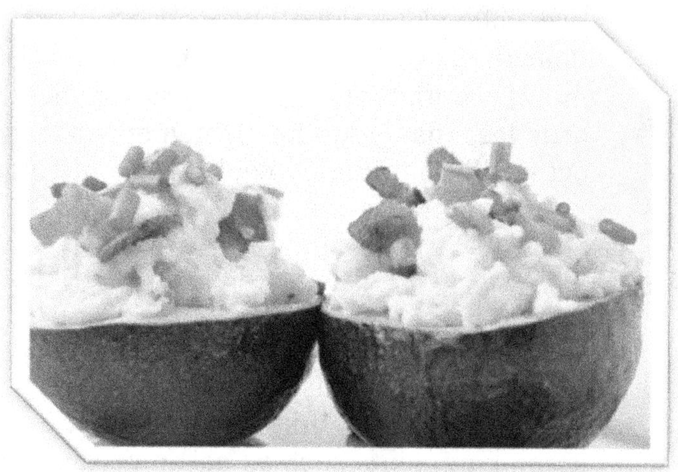

Prep time: 12 mins

4 portions

Ingredients

- Two eggs, hard
- ½ avocado
- 1 tsp olive oil
- 60 g bacon
- salt and pepper

Preparations

1. Preheat the oven to 180 ° C (350 ° F).
2. Put the eggs in a pot and cover with water. Bring to a boil and let simmer for 8-10

minutes. Place the eggs in ice water as soon as they are made to make it easier to peel them.

3. Split the eggs into two halves along and take out the yolks. Put them in a small bowl.
4. Add avocado and oil to the bowl and mash until mixed — salt and pepper to taste.
5. Place the bacon in a baking sheet and bake until crispy. Take 5-7 minutes. You can also fry them in a pan.
6. With a spoon, carefully add the mixture to the egg whites and place the bacon candle. To enjoy!

Tips

No doubt fun for children, but also fun for adults... also, these eggs are durable and nice enough to be your food in the basket.

Nutrition

Ketogenic low in carbons

Per portion

- Net carbohydrates: 2% (1 g)
- Fiber: 2 g
- Fat: 83% (13 g)
- Protein: 15% (5 g)
- kcal: 144

The Classic Bacon With Eggs

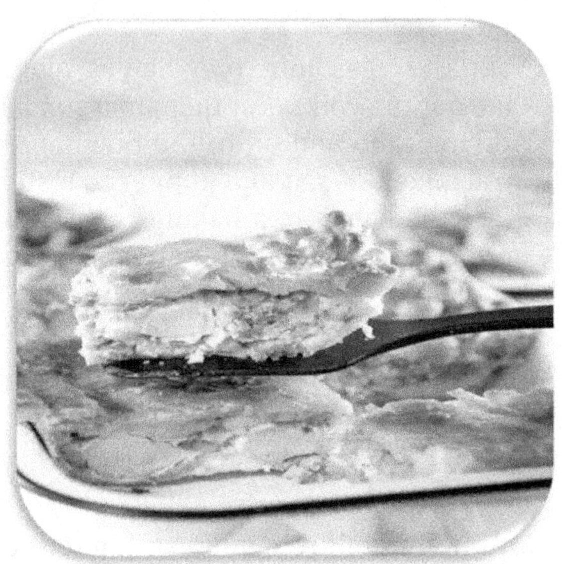

Prep time: 10 mins

4 portions

Ingredients

- Eight eggs
- 150 g bacon, sliced
- Cherry Tomatoes (optional)
- Fresh parsley (optional)

Preparations

Fry the bacon until crispy. Set aside on a plate.

Fry the eggs in the bacon fat the way you like. Cut the cherry tomatoes in half and fry them at the same time.

Salt and pepper to taste.

Tips

If you can, try using organic bacon... it's healthier and contains fewer additives.

Nutrition fact

Ketogenic low in carbons

Per portion

- Net carbohydrates: 2% (1 g)
- Fiber: 0 g
- Fat: 76% (23 g)
- Protein: 23% (16 g)
- Kcal: 282

Ketogenic Frittata Of Goat Cheese And Mushrooms

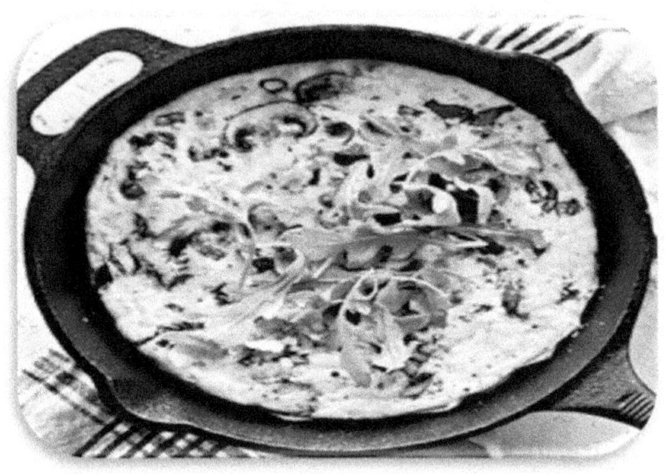

Prep time: 30 mins

2 portions

Ingredients

- Frittata
- 150 g mushrooms
- 75 g fresh spinach
- 50 g chives
- 50 g butter
- Six eggs
- 110 g goat cheese
- Salt and ground black pepper
- At your service
- 150 g green leafy vegetables

- 2 tbsp olive oil
- Salt and ground black pepper

Preparations

1. Preheat the oven to 175 ° C (350 ° F).
2. Grate or crumble the cheese and mix in a bowl with the eggs — salt and pepper to taste.
3. Cut the mushrooms into small pieces. Chop the chives.
4. 4. In an oven-fitting pan, melt the butter over medium heat and fry the mushrooms and onions for 5-10 minutes or until golden brown. Add the spinach to the pan and fry for another 1-2 minutes. Pepper.
5. Pour the egg mixture in the pan — Bake for about 20 minutes or until browned and firm in the middle.
6. Serve with green leafy vegetables and olive oil.

Scrambled Eggs In A Cup

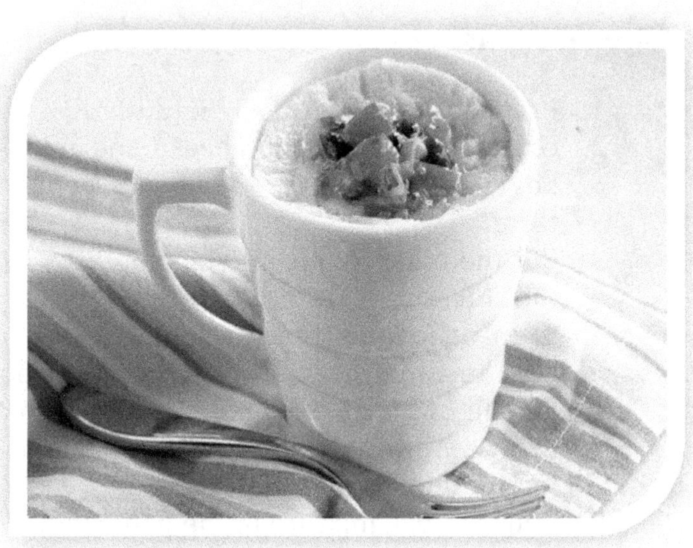

Prep time: 3 mins

1 portion

Ingredients

- Two eggs
- 2 tbsp cream to beat
- salt and pepper
- 1 tbsp Butter

Preparations

1. Grease a large cup or bowl with mild butter. Beat the eggs and the cream to beat. Fill the

cup to a maximum of two thirds, as the eggs will gain volume when cooked.

2. Add a pinch of salt and freshly ground black pepper or cayenne.

3. Cook in the microwave at maximum power for 1-2 minutes (700 watts). Stir and microwave another minute. Keep in mind that the eggs are still made after removing them from the heat, so do not overdo them.

4. Remove and add a little butter. Allow cooling for one minute.

Nutrition fact

Ketogenic low in carbons

Per portion

- Net carbohydrates: 2% (1 g)
- Fiber: 0 g
- Fat: 84% (31 g)
- Protein: 15% (12 g)
- kcal: 329

Keto Plate Of Turkey

Prep time: 5 mins

2 portions

Ingredients

- 175 g turkey cold cuts
- Two avocados
- 75 g (75 ml) cream cheese
- 50 g lettuce
- 60 ml of olive oil
- Salt or pepper

Preparations

1. Put the turkey, sliced avocado, lettuce and cream cheese on a plate.
2. Pour olive oil over the vegetables and season to taste.

Advice!

Do not hesitate to add a couple of sticks of celery and fill the hollow of the celery with cream cheese. Crisp!

Nutrition fact

Ketogenic low in carbons

Per portion

- Net carbohydrates: 4% (9 g)
- Fiber: 14 g
- Fat: 84% (75 g)
- Protein: 12% (24 g)
- Kcal: 820

Omelet Of Keto Cheese

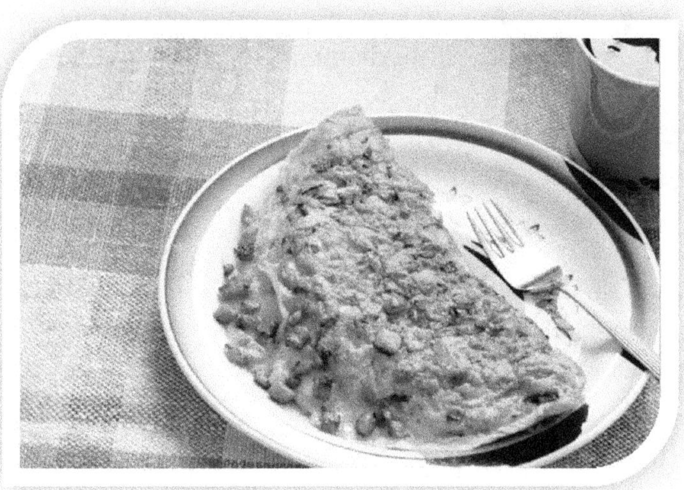

Prep time: 15 mins

2 portions

Ingredients

- 75 g butter
- Six eggs
- 200 g shredded cheddar cheese
- Salt and black pepper ground to taste

Preparations

1. Beat the eggs until soft and lightly frothy. Add half of the grated cheddar cheese and mix. Salt and pepper to taste.
2. Melt the butter in a hot pan. Pour the egg mixture and let stand for a few minutes.
3. Lower the heat and continue cooking until the egg mixture is almost done. Add the remaining grated cheese. Fold and serve immediately.

Advice!

Flavor your creation with herbs, chopped vegetables, or even Mexican sauce. And do not hesitate to cook the tortilla with olive oil or coconut oil to have a different flavor profile.

Nutrition fact

Ketogenic low in carbons

For portion

-   Net carbohydrates: 2% (4 g)
-   Fiber: 0 g
-   Fat: 81% (80 g)
-   Protein: 18% (40 g)
-   kcal: 897

Egg Muffins

Prep time: 25 mins

4 portions

Ingredients

- Eight eggs
- One spring onion, finely chopped
- 150 g dried chorizo with air or salami or cooked bacon
- 75 g grated cheese
- 1 tbsp red pesto or green pesto (optional)
- Salt and ground black pepper

Preparations

1. Preheat the oven to 175 ° C (350 ° F).
2. Chop the chives and meat finely.
3. Beat the eggs together with the condiments and the pesto. Add the cheese and mix.
4. Put the dough into muffin molds and add bacon, sausage or salami.
5. Bake for 15-20 minutes, depending on the size of the mold.

Tips!

Kids love these muffins full of cheese. They are perfect for carrying in the lunch box.

Coffee With Cream

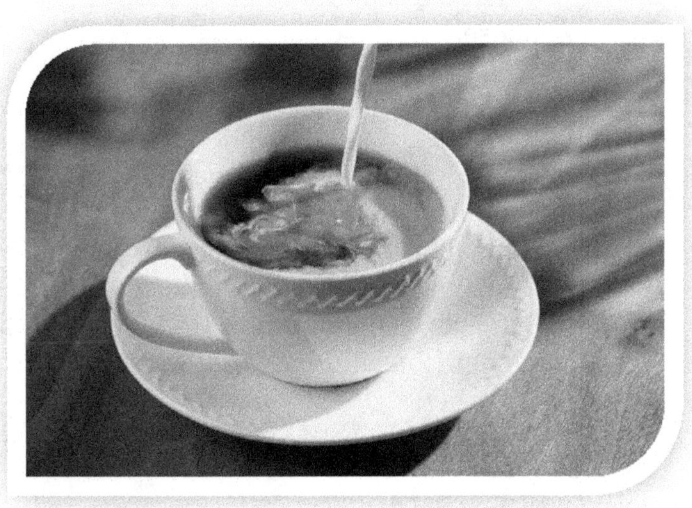

Prep time: 5mins

1 portion

Ingredients

- 180 ml coffee, prepared the way you like
- 60 ml whipping cream

Preparations

1. Prepare the coffee as you like. Pour the cream in a small saucepan and heat gently while stirring until frothy.

2. Pour the hot cream into a large cup, add the coffee and stir. Serve at the moment as it is or with a handful of nuts or a piece of cheese.

Tips

- Add a piece of dark chocolate with a minimum of 70% cocoa powder to your coffee cup. This way, you will have a little whim, waiting for when you finish drinking. Or try it with cinnamon to have a fabulous and delicious indulgence after the meal!

Nutrition fact

Ketogenic low in carbons

For portion

- Net carbohydrates: 3% (2 g)
- Fiber: 0 g
- Fat: 93% (22 g)
- Protein: 4% (2 g)
- Kcal: 207

CHAPTER 11

LUNCH RECIPES

If you want to have a balanced diet, it is necessary to know the basics of nutrition, the groups of foods that you must include, and the quantities. If you want to maintain your ideal weight and feel full of energy throughout the day, this is how your plate should look: 20-30g of protein; If you eat meat, a portion of your hand's palm should be the size. 8g of fiber in fruits, vegetables, and cereals. 50-65g of carbohydrates such as rice, bread, pasta, or legumes. 13-18g of fat, such as olive oil, walnuts or avocado. Finally, you should consume only 4g of sugars, preferably from the fruit.

Another important thing is to respect your schedule: try to eat lunch for about 3 hours after your morning snack.

Below you will find ideas of healthy, balanced, and very complete meals.

Greek Orzo Salad

Prep Time: 40 minutes

6 portions

Ingredients

Dressing

- 1/3 cup olive oil
- 3 Tbsp fresh lemon juice
- 1 clove garlic , minced
- Salt and freshly ground black pepper
- Salad
- ¼ cups (8 oz) dry orzo
- 1 cup (5 oz) crumbled feta
- 1 medium cucumber
- 1 (10.5 oz) pkg. grape tomatoes
- ½ cup sliced kalamata olives or 3/4 cup sliced black olives
- ½ cup chopped red onion, rinsed under water to removed harsh bite
- 3 Tbsp chopped fresh basil
- 2 Tbsp chopped fresh parsley

Instructions

1. In a jar mix together olive oil, lemon juice, garlic and season with salt and pepper to taste (don't add too much salt because the feta and kalamata olives are pretty salty), set aside.

2. Cook orzo according to directions listed on package. Drain and let cool (about 5 minutes. They'll start to stick to each other a bit but that's fine the dressing will break it up).
3. Add all of the salad ingredients, including cooked orzo, to a large bowl and toss. Pour dressing over top and toss to evenly coat. Store in refrigerator, serve within a few hours for best results.

Nutrition Facts

Amount Per Serving

Calories 320 Calories from Fat 171

- Total Fat 19g 29%
- Saturated Fat 5g 25%
- Cholesterol 22mg 7%
- Sodium 458mg 19%
- Potassium 199mg 6%
- Total Carbohydrates 28g 9%
- Dietary Fiber 1g 4%
- Sugars 3g
- Protein 8g 16%
- Vitamin A 8%
- Vitamin C 9.4%
- Calcium 15.1%
- Iron 5.3%

Tuna And Chickpea Pita Sandwiches

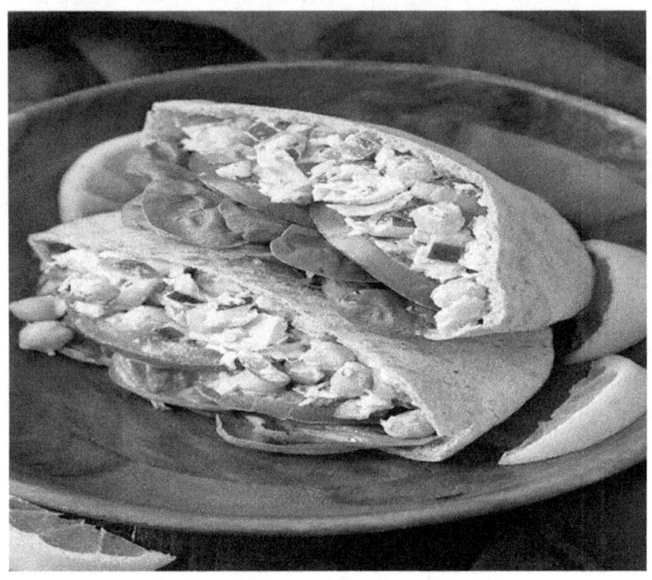

Prep Time: 30 minutes

4 portions

Ingredients

Dressing

- 1/3 cup fat-free or low-fat Greek yogurt
- ¼ cup light mayonnaise
- 2 1/2 Tbsp fresh lemon juice
- ¼ cup chopped fresh parsley
- 2 tsp chopped fresh rosemary or ½ tsp dried crushed

- 1tsp chopped fresh thyme leaves or ¼ tsp dried

Tuna Salad

- 2 (4.5 - 5 oz) cans white albacore tuna, drained well
- 1 (15 o) can chickpeas (aka garbanzo beans), drained and rinsed
- ¾ cup chopped celery
- 1/3 cup finely chopped red onion
- Salt and freshly ground black pepper
- 2 medium tomatoes, sliced
- 2 cups spinach
- 2 Whole wheat pita pocket breads

Instructions

1. In a small mixing bowl whisk together Greek yogurt, mayonnaise, lemon juice, parsley, and thyme or rosemary.
2. To a medium mixing bowl add tuna chickpeas, celery, and red onion. Pour Greek yogurt mixture over the top and toss everything to evenly coat.
3. Season with salt and pepper to taste and toss.
4. Slice pita pockets in half then slice through the center to open.
5. Layer in spinach, tomatoes and tuna salad mixture. Serve immediately.

Nutrition Facts

Amount Per Serving

Calories 321 Calories from Fat 72

% Daily Value*

- Total Fat 8g 12%
- Saturated Fat 1g 5%
- Cholesterol 31mg 10%
- Sodium 721mg 30%
- Potassium 659mg 19%
- Total Carbohydrates 36g 12%
- Dietary Fiber 8g 32%
- Sugars 3g
- Protein 23g 46%
- Vitamin A 42.9%
- Vitamin C 24%
- Calcium 10.7%
- Iron 19.8%

* Percent Daily Values are based on a 2000 calorie diet.

Mason Jar Chickpea, Farro And Greens Salad

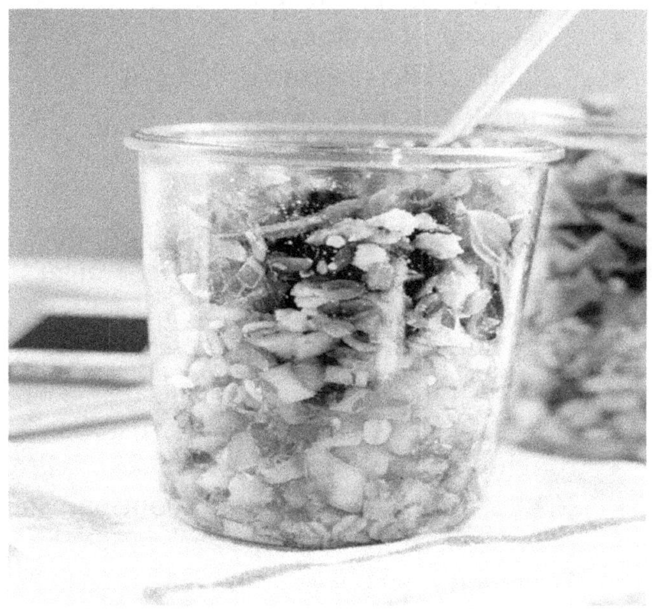

Prep Time: 1h:30 mins

4 portions

Ingredients

- Farro (feel free to substitute another grain and/or cook extra for later)
- 1 ¼ cup farro
- 1 tablespoon olive oil
- 1 medium clove garlic, pressed or minced
- ¼ teaspoon salt
- Greek dressing (this recipe is easily halved)

- 1 cup quality extra-virgin olive oil, such as California Olive Ranch brand
- ½ cup red wine vinegar
- 4 cloves garlic, pressed or minced
- 1 tablespoon dried oregano
- 2 teaspoons Dijon mustard
- 1 ½ teaspoons salt
- 1 teaspoon freshly ground black pepper
- 1 teaspoon agave nectar, honey or sugar
- Chickpea and celery salad
- 2 cans chickpeas (or 3 cups cooked chickpeas), drained and rinsed
- 4 stalks celery, thinly sliced crosswise and roughly chopped
- ⅔ cup chopped red onion (about one small red onion, chopped)
- 1 cup chopped parsley
- ⅓ cup Greek dressing or olive oil and lemon juice, to taste
- Greens and garnishes

Mixed greens, roughly chopped if you have time (a couple handfuls per salad)

- ¼ cup pepitas (pumpkin seeds) or sunflower seeds
- Handful dried cherries or cranberries, roughly chopped
- Kalamata olives, pitted and thinly sliced (optional)
- Feta cheese, crumbled (optional)

Preparation

1. To cook the farro: In a medium saucepan, combine the rinsed farro with at least three cups water (enough water to cover the farro by a couple of inches). Bring the water to a boil, then reduce heat to a gentle simmer, and cook until the farro is tender to the bite but still pleasantly chewy. (Pearled farro will take around 15 minutes, unprocessed farro will take 25 to 40 minutes.) Drain off the excess water and mix in the olive oil, garlic and salt. Set aside to cool.

2. Make the dressing: Whisk together all of the dressing ingredients until emulsified.

3. Make the chickpea and celery salad: In a serving bowl, toss together the chickpeas, prepared celery, red onion and parsley. Stir in enough dressing (or olive oil and lemon juice) to lightly coat the salad: Toss and set aside.

4. Toast the pepitas: In a skillet over medium-low heat, toast the pepitas for a few minutes, stirring frequently, until they smell fragrant and toasty. Transfer the pepitas to a bowl to cool.

5. To assemble your mason jar salads: In a quart-sized mason jar (32 ounce capacity), layer the chickpea salad at the bottom along with an additional tablespoon or two of dressing (enough to lightly coat the salad when you turn the jar upside down). Top

with cooled farro, then greens (leave about an inch of room at the top). Finish with a sprinkle of.

Nutrition Facts

Serves 4

Amount Per Serving

Calories 702

- Total Fat 28.6g 44%
- Saturated Fat 3.5g
- Trans Fat 0g
- Polyunsaturated Fat 7.8g
- Monounsaturated Fat 13.7g 0%
- Cholesterol 0mg 0%
- Sodium 534.6mg 22%
- Total Carbohydrate 92g 31%
- Dietary Fiber 21.2g 85%
- Sugars 15.2g
- Protein 22.8g 46%
- Vitamin A 11%
- Vitamin C 26%
- Calcium 20%
- Iron 38%
- Vitamin D 0%
- Magnesium 24%
- Potassium 21%
- Zinc 17%
- Phosphorus 34%

- Thiamin (B1) 15%
- Riboflavin (B2) 16%
- Niacin (B3) 10%
- Vitamin B6 55%
- Folic Acid (B9) 27%
- Vitamin B12 0%
- Vitamin E 4%
- Vitamin K 184%

Light Lunch

2 portions

Prep time: 15 mins

Ingredients

- 150g Beef fillet, thinly sliced
- 5 tbsp soy sauce
- 2 tbsp sherry
- 200g Sugar snap
- One teaspoon oil
- 1 Mango
- cayenne pepper
- 1 tbsp sesame
- salt

Preparation

1. Drill beef with soy sauce and sherry.
2. Clean the mangetouts and cut them into pieces — Cook in boiling and salted water for about 4 minutes and then drain.
3. Fry the meat in oil for a short time. Peel the mango and cut into small pieces. Add mango pieces together with the mangetouts and fry for a short time. Season with soy sauce and cayenne pepper serve and sprinkle with sesame seeds.
4. Serve with rice.

Cream - The Lunch

4 portions

Prep time: 45 mins

Ingredients

- 2 tbsp butter
- 2 tbsp Flour
- 200 ml of milk
- 500 ml of vegetable stock
- 2 tbsp tomato paste
- 200 ml of water
- 1 cup creme fraiche Cheese
- 500 g vegetables of your choice
- 500 g poultry meat, e.g., chicken breast
- 1 kg potato
- Salt and pepper as needed
- Vegetable oil for frying

Preparation

1. Peel potatoes, cook in salted water until cooked. Drain off water and briefly steam potatoes.
2. Cut the meat into large cubes and sauté in a little oil. Do the same with mushrooms and paprika. Wash broccoli and cauliflower, cook the florets in salted water until firm.
3. For the sauce, heat two tablespoons butter and stir in the flour. Deglaze the roux with the broth. Stir in tomato paste, milk, and

crème fraîche. Add the contents of the pan and the cooked vegetables. To prevent it from getting too thick, add the water as needed.

4. Arrange the plates with boiled potatoes and the cream and decorate with freshly ground colored pepper.

5. The dish was originally made with ready-made cream sauce, which was stirred into crème fraîche. A friend thought it was so delicious and wanted to know what it's called. When I said that it has no name, he said, it is now called "Cream."

6. As paprika, broccoli, cauliflower, but also mushrooms fit.

Super Easy Party – Ham

8 portions

Prep time: 15 mins

Ingredients

- 2kg Roast pork (crust roast), cured

Preparation

1. Preheat the oven to 220 °. Slice the rind into a diamond shape (carefully, do not cut into the meat), and wrap the crusty roast with the rind upwards in aluminum foil. The stewed crusted roast is usually spicy enough and does not need any further seasoning.
2. Bake the ham at 200 ° C on the middle rack for about 60 minutes. Then open the foil at the top and sprinkle the ham with the resulting gravy from time to time. Bake the ham for about 40 minutes.
3. After baking, cut the rind off the ham and cut the ham into thicker slices. Serve with sauerkraut and fried potatoes or simply delicious on a bread roll.

Custard With Quark And Fruit

12 portions

Prep time: 45 mins

Ingredients

- 1000 ml of milk
- 6 tbsp sugar
- Two-pack of pudding powder, vanilla
- 1 kg quark (lean quark)
- 4 tbsp sugar
- 1 point vanilla sugar
- 250 ml of milk
- 500 ml whipped cream
- 2 pts vanilla sugar
- 1kg fruit of your choice (cherries, strawberries, peaches, etc.)

Preparation

1. From the milk, the 6 tbsp sugar and the custard powder cook according to Preparations a custard and let cool. Cover it so that it does not form any skin.
2. Mix the quark with the four tablespoons of sugar, the vanilla sugar and the 250 ml of milk.
3. Beat the cream with the vanilla sugar until stiff.
4. Prepare fruit, corer according to variety, cut small.

5. Once the pudding has cooled, stir in the cottage cheese. Then fold in the whipped cream and the fruit.
6. (Depending on your taste, sweeten!)
7. Again cold for a while and then enjoy!

Nutrition Facts

Amount Per Serving

Calories 600 Calories from Fat 310

% Daily Value*

- Total Fat 34.4g 53%
- Saturated Fat 5.9g 30%
- Sodium 1435mg 60%
- Potassium 923mg 26%
- Total Carbohydrates 54.7g 18%
- Dietary Fiber 10.1g 40%
- Sugars 9.7g
- Protein 20.7g 41%
- Calcium 33%
- Iron 77%

* Percent Daily Values are based on a 2000 calorie diet.

Exotic Tuna - Sauce To Rice

3 portions

Prep time: 10 mins

Ingredients

- One can tuna
- One can Pineapple slices
- 2 m. - Large onion
- 200 ml of coconut milk
- 50 ml broth
- 1 tbsp Oil (peanut, sunflower or sesame oil)
- ½ EL butter
- 1 tbsp Curry or
- Curry paste, red
- 1 tbsp. Flour
- Salt and pepper, whiter, ground

Preparation

1. The onions are first halved from top to bottom, then sliced lengthwise into thin slices and sautéed in oil and butter over low heat for 5 minutes. Then the drained tuna is added and fried.
2. Mix with curry and flour, continue for a short time. Add the broth and top up with the coconut milk. Simmer briefly, add the sliced pineapple (two slices or to taste) and season with salt, pepper and a good dash of pineapple juice.
3. Serve with rice.

CHAPTER 12

SNACK RECIPES

Delicious Cinnamon Stars With Nutri-Plus Hazelnut

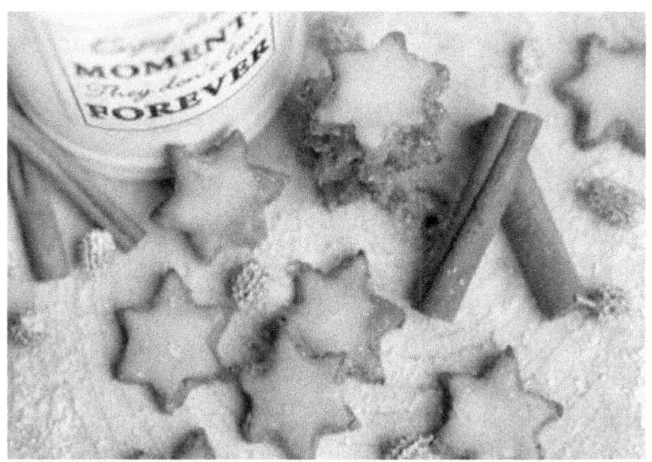

Prep time: 45 mins

3 portions

Ingredients

- 150g Almonds, ground
- 200g Ground hazelnuts
- 60g Coconut blossom sugar
- 60g Nutri-Plus Shape & Shake Hazelnut

- 3 tsp cinnamon
- 5g Orange peel, abrasion
- 15g Chia seeds
- 120 ml of water
- One pinch of salt
- 100g xylitol
- One lemon

Preparation

1. Stir the chia seeds into the water and let it swell slightly.
2. Put all the other ingredients, except for xylitol and lemon juice, together in a bowl and mix thoroughly.
3. Now you can add the water with the chia seeds and knead everything together.
4. Roll the dough into a ball and wrap it in cling film. Put it in the fridge for about an hour.
5. Roll the dough out about one centimeter thick and cut out little stars.
6. Repeat that until no dough is left.
7. Preheat the oven to 170 ° C and let the stars bake for about 8-10 minutes.
8. Get your stars out of the oven and let them cool.
9. Then stir the icing from small ground xylitol and lemon juice and decorate your cinnamon stars.

Nutrition fact

Values per serving

- Calories for cinnamon star 55 kcal
- Fat 3.5 g
- carbohydrates 3.5 g
- protein 2 g

Low Carb Poppy Seed Cake

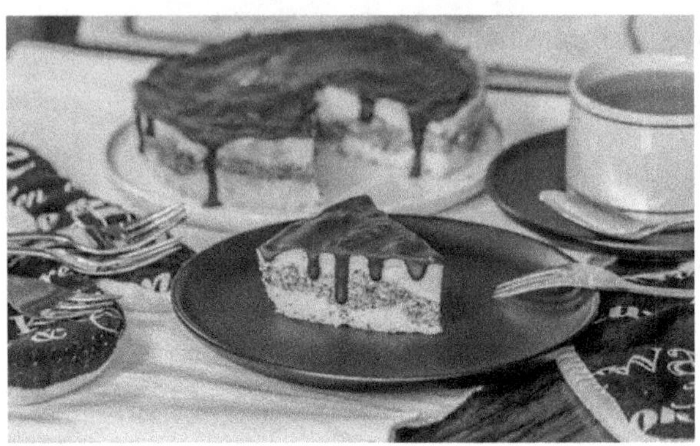

Prep time: 20 mins

3 portions

Ingredients

- 1000g Soy quark (Alpro or Provamel)
- Something Egg substitute for three eggs
- 75g protein powder vanilla
- 3 tbsp semolina
- One pack Custard powder (unsweetened)
- 3 tsp liquid sweetener or sugar light (about 4-5 tbsp)
- Quantity depending on the desired intensity Poppy

Preparation

1. Mix the egg mixture according to Preparation in a large bowl.
2. Add all remaining ingredients and stir the

cream with a hand mixer.

3. Place 1/3 of the mass in a separate bowl and stir in the poppy seeds (amount depending on the desired intensity of the poppy flavor.)
4. Place the mixed layer by layer in a baking or casserole dish lined with baking paper and bake at 200 ° C (top/bottom heat) or 180 ° C (circulating air) in a preheated oven for about 60 minutes.
5. The baking or casserole dish should not exceed 20 cm in diameter. Otherwise, the cake is too flat.
6. After baking, allow to cool (preferably in the fridge overnight) and glaze with melted dark chocolate.

Nutrition fact

Values for serving

- Calories apiece 112
- Carbohydrates 3 g
- Protein 12 g
- Fat 6

Refreshing Blueberry Bites

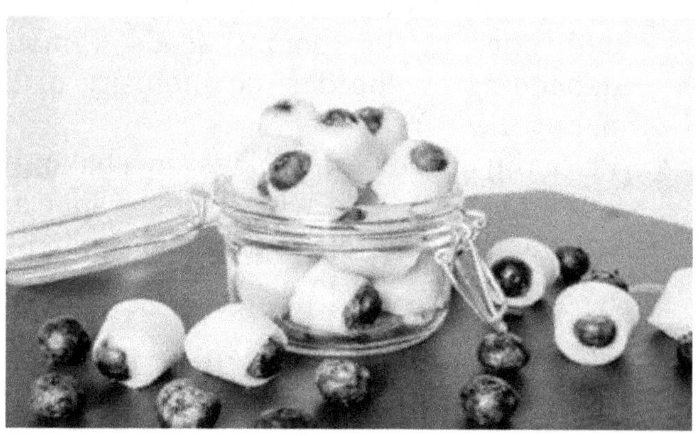

Prep time: 5 mins

2 portions

Ingredients

- 24 blueberries
- 250g soy yogurt, unsweetened
- 20g protein powder, lemon cake

Preparation

1. You need 1-2 ice cube
2. Molds for a total of 24 yogurt bites.
3. Wash the blueberries and place each blueberry in a tray of ice cubes.
4. Stir the yogurt together with the protein powder until no more lumps are visible.

5. Carefully pour the yogurt into the ice cubes and place them in the freezer overnight.
6. Snacking is allowed at any time

Nutrition facts

values per serving

- Calories per bite 9 kcal
- Fat 0.25 g
- Carbohydrates 0.2 g
- Protein 1 g

Chia Protein Energy Balls

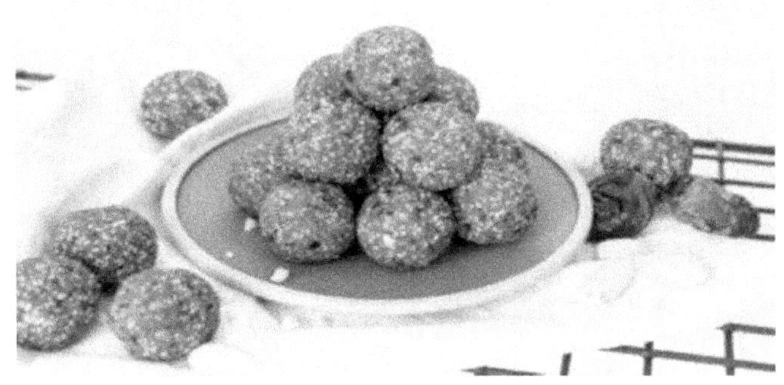

Prep time: 15 mins

Portions: 18 energy balls

Ingredients

- 60g ground almonds
- 60g chopped almonds
- 60g chia seeds
- 20g protein powder chocolate
- 120g dates

Preparation

1. Soak the dates in a little water for at least 15 minutes.
2. Add the softened dates, almonds, Chia seeds, and protein powder in a powerful blender.
3. Mix everything properly until a dough is formed.

4. Moisten your hands a little and then take about 1 tsp of dough per ball from the blender.
5. Roll the dough between your hands into small balls.
6. Optionally roll the balls in a topping of your choice. Coconut flakes, cocoa powder, chopped nuts... everything is possible.

Store the finished balls in the refrigerator.

Nutrition facts

Values for serving

Calories per ball, 81 kcal

Fat 5 g

Carbohydrates 5 g

Protein 3 g

Protein Bars For The Extra Portion Of The Power

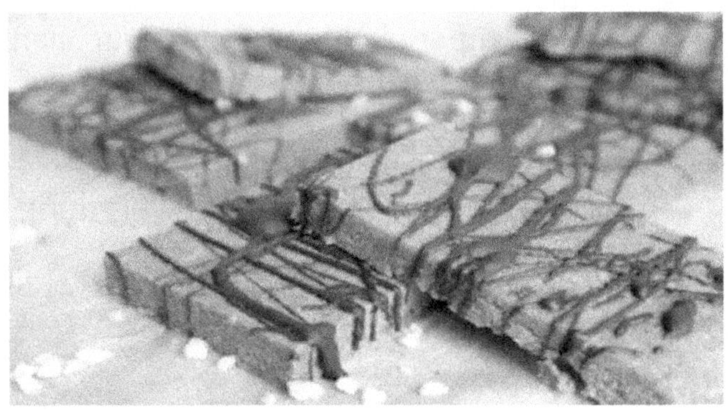

Prep time: 15 mins

Portions: 8 bars

Ingredients

- 90g protein powder vanilla
- 30g coconut flower syrup
- 100g chopped almonds
- 70g Cashewmus
- 10g coconut oil
- 50ml water
- One pinch salt
- Optional cinnamon

Preparation

1. You can put all the ingredients directly into a strong blender and mix until a nice firm consistency is created.

2. Put out the mold with cling film.
3. Press the mass with your hands into the mold, and with a spoon, everything nice flat.
4. Put the mold in the fridge for at least one hour and let it set.
5. Remove the mold from the refrigerator and cut the bars into eight equal pieces.

Optional:

- Melt 30 g of dark chocolate in a water bath and gently pour over the finished bars.

Nutrition fact

Values for serving

- Calories for bar 190 kcal
- Fat 12 g
- Carbohydrates 7 g
- Protein 14 g

Mango Nice Cream

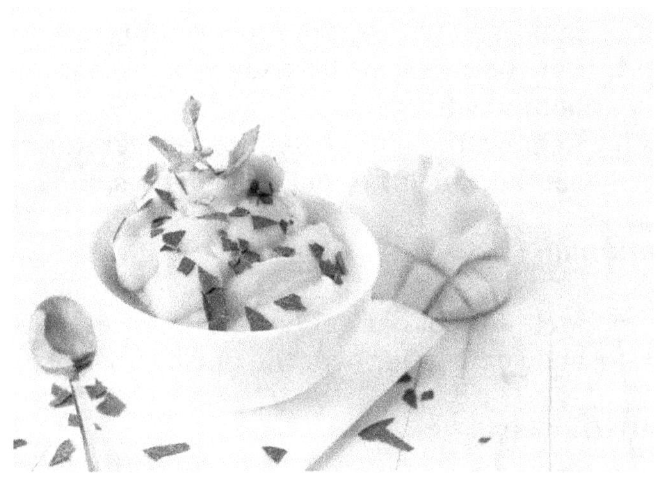

Prep time: 10 mins

1 portion

Ingredients

- Two frozen bananas
- One ripe mango
- 30g protein powder vanilla
- 30ml vegetable milk
- Something mint
- Something grated chocolate

Preparation

1. The bananas are best frozen one day before cut into small pieces.

2. Put the bananas, the mango, the protein powder, and the soy milk together in a blender and stir until creamy.
3. Then top with mint and chocolate grated.

Sweet Hummus Dip For Snacking

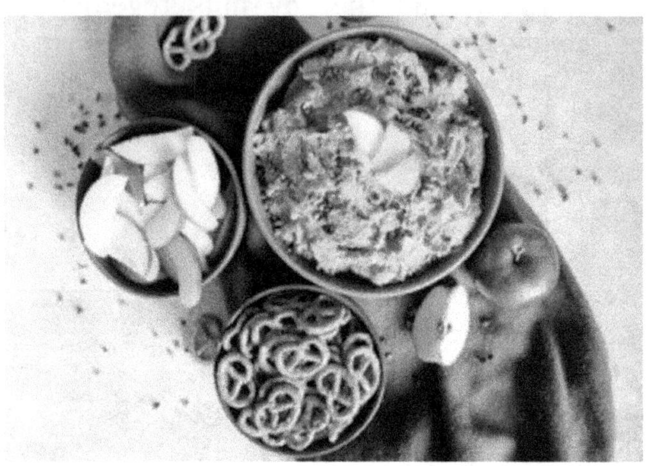

Prep time: 10 minutes

2 portions

Ingredients

- 480g Chickpeas (canned)
- 40g protein powder chocolate
- 30g agave nectar
- 60g Peanut butter
- 100 ml of soy milk
- 2 Teaspoons cinnamon
- One vanilla bean
- One pinch salt

Preparation

Results in about 600 g

1. Wash the chickpeas from the can thoroughly under running water.
2. Remove the marrow from the vanilla pod and then add all ingredients to a powerful blender.
3. Mix the mass until a homogeneous cream is produced.
4. Fill the sweet hummus in a bowl, and you can already enjoy a snack.

TIP: Sweet or salty, you can dive pretty much anything you want.

- Our hummus dip is also suitable as a sweet spread or to pimp on the porridge.

Nutrition fact

Values for Serving

- Calories for 100 g 170 kcal
- Fat 6 g
- Carbohydrates 15 g
- Protein 13 g

High-Protein Pizza Cabbage

Prep time: 30 mins

4 Portion

Ingredients

- 200g spelled flour
- 60g neutral protein powder
- 200 ml of water
- 10g baking powder
- 100 ml Sieved tomatoes
- 1 tbsp mixed herbs
- 80g colorful paprika
- 30g mushrooms
- 30g peas
- 20g olives
- One spring onion
- Smoothing of salt, pepper, paprika

Preparation

1. Preheat the oven to 180 ° C.
2. Put the spilled flour, the protein powder, the baking powder, and a pinch of salt in a bowl and mix everything thoroughly.
3. Now add the water and knead the mass into a firm dough.
4. Divide the dough into four pieces to form flat baguettes.

5. Place the baguettes on a baking sheet lined with baking paper and bake for about 5 minutes.
6. In time you take care of the surface. Mix the tomato with herbs and spices and cut the vegetables into small cubes.
7. Remove the pre-baked baguettes from the oven, sprinkle with the tomato sauce and spread the toppings on top.
8. Bake the pizza cabbies for another 10 minutes until they are nicely brown and crispy.

Nutritional values for serving

- Calories for pizza baguette 265 kcal
- Fat 2 g
- Carbohydrates 40 g
- Protein 20 g

Energy Balls Made From Chickpeas

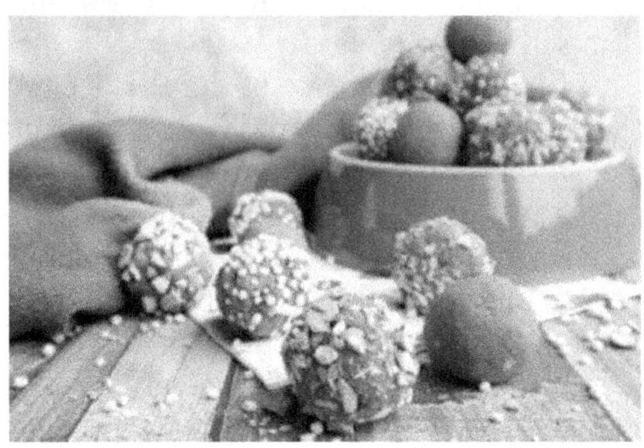

Prep time: 45 minutes

Make 20 Energy Ball

Ingredients

- 90g oatmeal
- 30g Shape & Shake gingerbread
- 200g Chickpeas
- 50g dates (Medjoul)
- 20g cocoa powder
- One teaspoon cinnamon
- One pinch salt
- 100 ml of water

Preparation

1. Put the oatmeal in a blender and mash to flour.

2. Wash the chickpeas very thoroughly and then add them to the blender.
3. Remove the dates and add them to the blender along with all other ingredients.
4. Let the mixer do the rest of the work and turn the mass into a solid dough.
5. Take one teaspoon of dough and roll it into a ball between your hands.

Optional:

1. You can still roll the balls after rolling in a topping of your choice.
2. Quinoa, nuts, chia seeds, cocoa powder... everything is possible.

Tip:

- The cleaner you work, the longer the balls will last longer in the fridge.
- Wear gloves best when rolling.
- It does not have to be our Shape & Shake in the taste Gingerbread!
- Vanilla, hazelnut, or chocolate are also great.

Nutrition fact

Values for serving

- Calories for ball, 40 kcal
- Fat 0.8 g
- Carbohydrates 6 g
- Protein 3 g

The Healthy Fruit Bread For Snacking

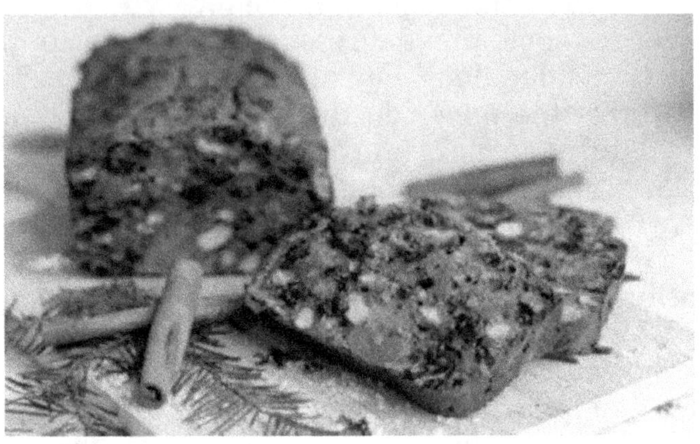

Prep time: 90 mins

3 portions

Ingredients

- 100g dried apricots
- 150g raisins
- 125g dried cranberries
- 2cm ginger
- 500ml apple juice
- One teaspoon of lemon peels, abrasion
- 500ml Apple juice, naturally cloudy
- 100g walnuts
- 50g pistachios
- 50g chopped almonds
- 50g protein powder vanilla
- 300g spelled flour
- 2 Teaspoon cinnamon

- ½ tsp cardamom
- One parcel baking powder

Preparations

Make a fruitcake of 1400 g

1. Cut the dried fruits into small pieces and put them together with the apple juice in a large bowl.
2. Grate the ginger, peel off the lemon zest and add both into the bowl.
3. Let it all stand for at least 30 minutes and pull through.
4. Chop the nuts, roughly and mix them with the spices, the protein powder, and the baking powder.
5. Add the mixture to the dried fruit and the apple juice and mix everything.
6. The typed flour is coming now. Slowly stir the flour bit by bit so that no lumps are formed.
7. Preheat the oven to 180 ° C and layout a baking pan with baking paper.
8. Put the mass in the pan and let the bread bake for 50-60 minutes.
9. Get it out of the oven and let it cool down a bit.
10. At best, lukewarm!
11. If the fruit bread becomes too dark when baking,
12. Cover it with a little aluminum foil.

Nutrition fact

Values for serving

- Calories for 100g /280 kcal
- Fat 9 g
- Carbohydrates 40 g
- Protein 9 g

CHAPTER 13

DINNER RECIPES

Zucchini Noodles With Avocado Cream And Tomatoes

Prep time: 10 minutes

2 portions

Ingredients

- 400g zucchini
- One avocado
- 100g cherry tomatoes
- 10g sesame
- 5g olive oil
- One clove of garlic
- 2-3 basil stems
- One pinch each salt and pepper

Preparation

1. Cut the zucchini into the pasta with a spiral cutter or peeler.
2. Peel a garlic clove and add it to the avocado along with the olive oil and some basil.
3. Puree the ingredients to a creamy mass.
4. Quarter the cherry tomatoes and put them under the avocado cream.
5. Season with salt and pepper and mix with the zucchini noodles.

6. Sprinkle with sesame and enjoy

TIP: If you do not tolerate raw zucchini so well, you can fry them briefly in a pan.

Nutritional facts

Values for serving

- Calories 450 kcal
- Carbohydrates 15 g
- Protein 10 g
- Fat 35 g

Vegan Fitness Kebab

Prep time: 20 mins

1 portion

Ingredients

- 1/2 packet Vegan Döner (brand "Wheaty")
- 75 g Parboiled Rice
- 2 tomatoes
- 1.2 onions
- 150g lettuce
- 150g soy yogurt (brand "Alpro")
- Something fresh herbs and spices
- Maybe something olive oil

Preparation

1. Wash the lettuce, tomatoes, and onion thoroughly and cut into small pieces. Meanwhile, cook the rice
2. Roast the vegan doner, he must be nice and crispy
3. Put the rice portion together with the salad, the tomatoes and the onions on a plate
4. Season the soy yogurt with fresh herbs and spices (maybe some olive oil) and pour over the salad
5. Finally, spread the fried vegan doner over it and season with some kebab seasoning

Nutritional facts

Values for serving

- Calories 680 kcal
- Fat 19 g
- Carbohydrates 78g
- Protein 44 g

Gluten-Free Chickpea Soup

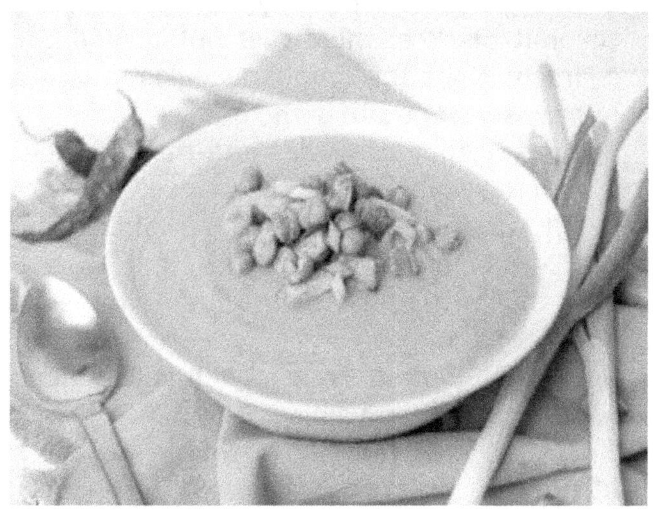

Prep time: 20 mins

1 portion

Ingredients

- 1 red onion
- 2 Garlic cloves
- 500g sweet potatoes
- 400g Chickpeas, cooked
- 1cm ginger
- 1l vegetable stock
- 30g neutral protein powder, gluten-free
- About 1 tsp Salt, pepper, turmeric, nutmeg
- One teaspoon of coconut oil

Preparation

1. First, remove the shell from the onion, garlic, and ginger, slice it roughly, and fry it in a little coconut oil. Peel the sweet potato and cut it coarsely. Once the onions are glassy, you can put the sweet potato in the pot.
2. Stew everything together and then extinguish it with the vegetable broth.
3. Let it simmer for about 10-12 minutes until the sweet potato is tender enough, then add the chickpeas. Let everything simmer for another 5 minutes.
4. Get the soup off the stove. Then take a blender and puree the soup a bit.
5. Now add the protein powder and let the blender do the rest of the work. Mix the soup until no pieces are left. Season with the spices and enjoy.
6. If you like, then you can roast some chickpeas and add to the soup as a topping.

Nutritional fact

Values for serving

- Calories for serving 550 kcal
- Carbohydrates 90 g
- Fat 9 g
- Protein 38 g

Protein Gnocchi With Basil Pesto

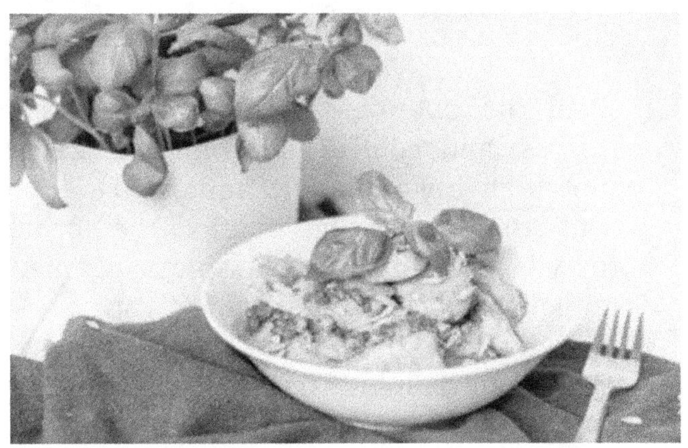

Prep time: 30 mins

4 portions

Ingredients

- 400g Potatoes, boiling
- 60g neutral protein powder
- 50g wheat flour
- ½ tsp salt
- Something nutmeg
- 2 tbsp Flour for the work surface
- One bunch of basil
- 30g pine nuts
- clove of garlic
- 100ml olive oil
- Something of salt and pepper

Preparation

The recipe is a bit tricky. So take your time.

1. Peel the potatoes, slice them into small pieces, and cook 20-25 minutes. Let the potatoes cool off !! (very important)
2. Put the pieces of potato, the protein powder, the flour, and the spices together in a blender and mix everything properly. The dough should have about the consistency of firm cake dough. If necessary, add flour or water.
3. Spread some flour on the work surface and divide the dough into four parts.
4. Moisten your hands to prevent the dough from sticking to your fingers and form long, round snakes out of the dough.
5. Slice the snakes every 1.5-2 cm, press briefly with a fork to keep the pesto better, and you're done with the raw gnocchi.
6. Now put the gnocchi together in lightly boiling water for 3-4 minutes and wait until they float up. Then they are done.

Now the pesto:

- Wash the basil thoroughly
- Add the basil, pine nuts, garlic, and olive oil to the blender.
- Mix all ingredients until a creamy consistency is achieved.

- Season with salt and pepper and serve directly with the gnocchi.

Nutritional facts

Values for serving

Calories for serving 860 kcal

Fat 55 g

Carbohydrates 55 g

Protein 35 g

Vegan Rosemary Roulade With Potatoes, Broccoli And Mushroom Sauce

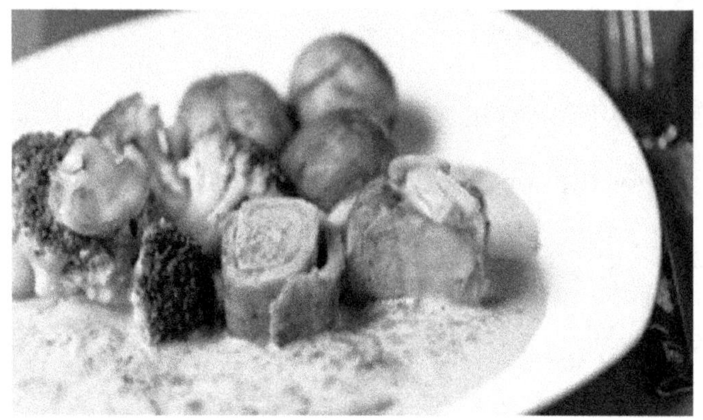

Prep time: 20 mins

2 portions

Ingredients

- 200g potatoes
- 200g broccoli
- 200g mushrooms
- 2 Rosemary-Vegan roulades
- 150 ml of plant milk
- 1.2 onion
- 10 g rye flour
- 1 tbsp safflower oil
- Something of salt and pepper

Preparations

1. Prepare the potatoes according to your preference (salt or jacket potatoes)
2. Meanwhile, cook the broccoli in salted water for about 10 minutes
3. Clean the mushrooms and the onions, cut and fry in a pan for about 10 minutes over medium heat (in case of danger that the whole thing burns, please fill with a little water)
4. Add the vegetable milk after the mushrooms and onions have softened, and bring to a boil. Simmer a little and bind with the flour, then season with salt and pepper.
5. Roast the rosemary and vegan roulades in a pan with a little oil on each side for about 2 minutes until golden brown
6. Serve on the plate and enjoy

Nutrition fact

values for serving

- Calories 403 kcal
- Fat 18 g
- Carbohydrates 25 g
- Protein 33 g

Protein Rice Pudding

Prep time: 7 mins

1 portion

Ingredients

- 150-200ml Oatmeal or other vegetable milk
- 30g Shape & Shake Protein Powder Vanilla
- 2-3 tbsp cooked rice
- Something of cinnamon and sugar light to sprinkle

Preparation

- Shake oat milk with protein powder in a shaker or blender.
- Mix with rice and warm in the microwave for a short time. But it also tastes cold.
- In the end, sprinkle with the cinnamon and sugar light mixture.

Vegan Sliced À La Bombay

Prep time: 25 minutes

2 portions

Ingredients

- 100g Vegan roast piece (brand "Wheaty")
- 75g Parboiled Rice
- 100g broccoli
- 150g pineapple
- 1. 4 onion
- 100ml of coconut milk
- Something of curry, pepper and vegetable broth
- Maybe something Locust bean gum

Preparation

1. Cook the rice
2. Chop the vegan roast and sauté
3. For the sauce, fry the onion and deglaze with coconut milk
4. Add the broccoli and cook
5. Season the sauce with curry, pepper and some vegetable stock (if the sauce is too liquid, you can use some carob seed flour)
6. In the end, add the pieces of pineapple (unsweetened) to the sauce

Nutrition fact

values for serving

- Calories 790 kcal
- Fat 27 g
- Carbohydrates 95 g
- Protein 37 g

Summery Bowls With Fresh Vegetables And Protein Quark

Prep time: 10 mins

2 portions

Ingredients

- 100g green salad
- 100g radish
- 200g kohlrabi
- 70g carrots
- 70g red lenses
- 50g tomatoes
- Two spring onions
- 20g Nuts / seeds
- 150g soy yogurt
- 2 tbsp mixed herbs
- One teaspoon of lemon juice
- 20g Shape & Shake, neutral
- One pinch salt, pepper

Preparation

1. Wash the salad and the vegetables and peel the kohlrabi.
2. Simmer the red lentils for about 7 minutes.
3. In time, cut/grate the vegetables.
4. Mix the soy yogurt with the lemon juice, the protein powder, some salt / pepper, and the herbs.

5. Arrange all ingredients together in a deep plate or bowl and top with the spring onions and nuts/seeds.

Nutritional fact

Values for serving

- Calories 630 kcal
- Fat 15 g
- Carbohydrates 60 g
- Protein 55 g

Crispy Asparagus Tart

Prep time: 30 minutes

Ingredients

- 150g spelled flour
- 30g Shape & Shake Neutral
- 130ml water
- 8 g dry yeast
- 1/2 tsp salt
- 200g soybean curd
- 2 tbsp mixed herbs
- One teaspoon lemon juice
- 200g green asparagus
- 100g cherry tomatoes
- 1 red onion
- 20 g pine nuts
- Smoothing Salt, pepper, chili flakes

Preparation

1. Beginning with the dough!
2. Put the flour, our protein powder, the yeast, and the salt in a bowl and mix all the dry ingredients thoroughly.
3. Second Now add the lukewarm water and knead everything together to a firm dough.
4. Leave the dough to rest for at least 30 minutes, taking care of the remaining ingredients over time.

5. Stir in the herb quark: Add the soy quark, the herbs, the lemon juice, and some salt to a bowl and stir together.
6. Then wash the asparagus and the tomatoes and cut both small.
7. Peel the onion and cut into fine rings.
8. Put some flour on the work surface and roll out the dough as thin as possible.
9. Spread the herb quark on the flame cake batter and spread the remaining ingredients on it.
10. Put the tarot cake in the preheated oven for about 10-12 minutes at 200 ° C.
11. Finally, sprinkle the pine nuts on the tarot cake and taste it.

Nutritional values for serving

- Calories 975 kcal
- Fat 25 g
- Carbohydrates 125 g
- Protein 65 g

Protein-Rich Asparagus Cream Soup

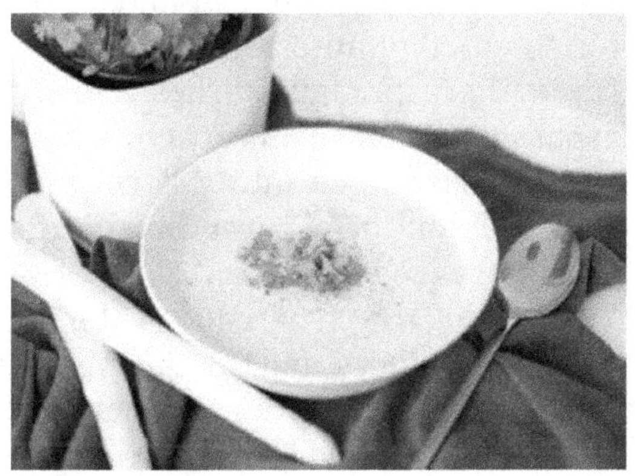

Prep time: 45 mins

Ingredients

- 1kg white asparagus
- 50g Alsan
- 40g spelled flour
- 1.2 l water
- 200ml of soy milk
- 30g neutral protein powder
- 1 punch each of salt, sugar, pepper and nutmeg
- 1.2 lemons
- Fresh parsley

Preparation

1. You should wash the asparagus thoroughly and cut off the woody, dry ends.

2. Peel the asparagus and cook the skins in the water with a pinch of salt and a little sugar for about 20 minutes.
3. Drain the asparagus dishes and catch the asparagus water in an extra bowl.
4. Cut the asparagus into 2-3 cm pieces and cook them in the asparagus water for about 15 minutes soft.
5. Then pour the asparagus water with the asparagus pieces and let the Alsen melt in the pot. Once the Alsen has melted, add the flour and gradually add a little bit of asparagus water until the whole liquid is used up.
6. Now mix the soymilk with the protein powder and put the shake in the pot. Let the soup simmer a bit, but do not boil properly!
7. Now you can put the asparagus pieces, the lemon juice, and the spices back into the soup and season to taste.
8. With fresh parsley, Serve and enjoy.

Nutritional fact

values for serving

- Calories per serving 430 kcal
- Fat 22g
- Carbohydrates 28g
- Protein 30g

CHAPTER 14

VEGETABLE RECIPES

Boar Stew With Vegetables, Herbs And Plums, A Tuscan Recipe

Prep time: 30 mins

4 portions

Ingredients

- 1kg wild boar from the club without fat and bone
- 1 onion
- 2 pole/s celery
- 1 carrot
- 5 Juniper berries
- 1 Garlic cloves
- 1 branch/s rosemary
- One branch/s Marjoram or dried rubbed
- 1 branch/s thyme
- ¾ liters of red wine, (Chianti)
- 60ml vinegar, (red wine vinegar)
- 3 tbsp flour
- 30g pine nuts
- Some prunes
- 30g chocolate, bitter, grated
- 6 tbsp olive oil
- salt
- Balsamic vinegar

Preparation

1. Cut the wild boar meat into cubes of about the same size and place it in a bowl. Add the wine, the sliced onion, celery, and carrot bits, crumbled bay leaf, crushed juniper berries, marjoram, thyme, crushed garlic, and rosemary. Cover with the marinade and let it simmer for 24 hours, stirring several times.

2. Remove the pieces of meat, drain, dab, and turn in the flour. Remove vegetables and herbs with a slotted spoon from the marinade and set aside.

3. Heat the oil in a saucepan and sauté the vegetables and herbs from the marinade. Take out and sear the meat well in the hot fat from all sides. Add the vegetables and herbs and deglaze with the marinade — cover and stew for about 3 hours on the lowest heat setting.

4. After 1 ½ hour, remove the meat with a slotted spoon and place on a plate. Fish the herb sprigs from the sauce and purée the gravy carefully with a wand. Put the meat and sauce back in the pot. Add the finely chopped pine nuts; the prunes cut into fine strips and the dark chocolate. Pour in the red wine vinegar and stew for another 1 ½ hours — season with some balsamic vinegar and salt.

Turkish ACMA With Sheep's Cheese And Vegetables

Typical Turkish recipe for a delicious breakfast

Prep time: 60 mins

6 portions

Ingredients

For the dough:

- 100ml of water
- 100ml of milk
- 100ml of oil
- 200g quark
- 1 tbsp salt
- 3 tbsp sugar
- Two pack Yeast, fresh
- 100ml cream
- 700g flour
- One pack baking powder

For the filling:

- 200g feta cheese
- ½ Bund parsley

For the decoration:

- 10 Cherry tomato
- Two peppers
- 10 olives

Also:

- One egg yolk

Preparation

1. For the dough, mix all the liquid ingredients. Mix the flour and baking powder, add gradually, and prepare the dough. Leave the dough in a warm place for 45 minutes.
2. Form small balls from the dough, brushing the hands with oil. Layout a baking tray with baking paper and place the balls over it. Cover your hands with oil now and then. Make a recess with your fingers in the balls and fill them with sheep's cheese and parsley. Decorate with tomatoes, peppers, and olives and let the balls go for another 15 minutes.
3. Brush with egg yolks and bake in a preheated oven at 160° C for 20 - 25 minutes.

My Creamy, Vegan Peanut Fritters With Vegetables And Soy

Vegan recipe (of course vegetarian)

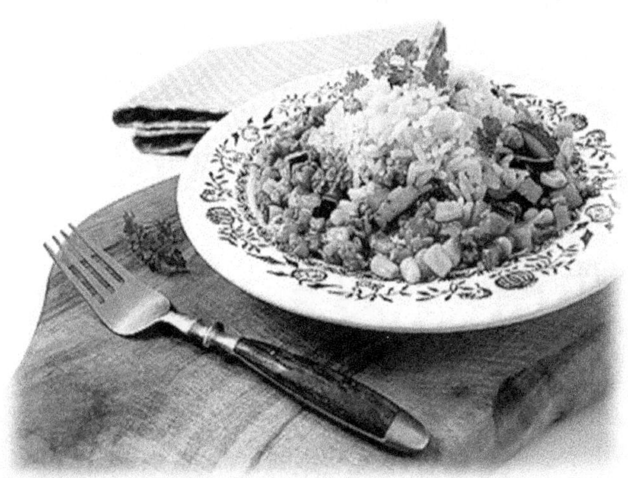

Prep time: 55 mins

Two portions

Ingredients

- ¾ cup soya granules
- Vegetable broth, hot, for soaking
- 1 m. Large Onion (s), diced
- 1 Garlic clove (s), crushed
- ½ m.-large Carrot (s), diced
- ½ m.-large Zucchini, diced
- One can Corn, (or 140g vegetable corn)
- 100ml Vegetable stock, strong

- 150ml of Soy milk (soy drink)
- 3 tbsp soy sauce
- 3 tbsp peanut butter
- 1 tbsp parsley
- Something chili powder
- Something pepper
- Possibly. Curry powder
- Possibly. Paprika
- Something vegetable oil, for searing
- Possibly. Flour, to thicken

Preparation

1. Soy granules in a bowl. Bring the vegetable stock to a boil and pour over the granules. It should not be in the "dry" and swell well. Let it swell for at least 5 minutes. Then express properly and possibly season with a little salt or broth (can taste nice strong).
2. Heat vegetable oil in the pan and add the granules. The best taste is achieved, in my opinion, if you let the granules neatly burn until it is nicely browned and crispy.
3. Then add the diced onions, carrots, and the crushed garlic clove and also lightly brown.
4. Finally, add the diced zucchini and corn.
5. Add the mixture of soymilk, vigorous vegetable broth, and soy sauce.
6. The peanut butter (I like it very creamy and add four tablespoons), add pepper and chili powder.

7. Cover and simmer everything until the zucchini are done. If it has become too thick, add some soy milk or water.
8. Finally, to taste again.
9. The sauce should be nice creamy with a good spiciness and seasoning.
10. If necessary, add a little broth, salt, chili powder or pepper. If you like it even thicker, with some flour, of course, you can also thicken.
11. Also, there is rice for me. If you like, you can also choose the other side dishes.
12. Some fresh parsley provides the last whistle.

Bolognese Sauce With Lots Of Vegetables

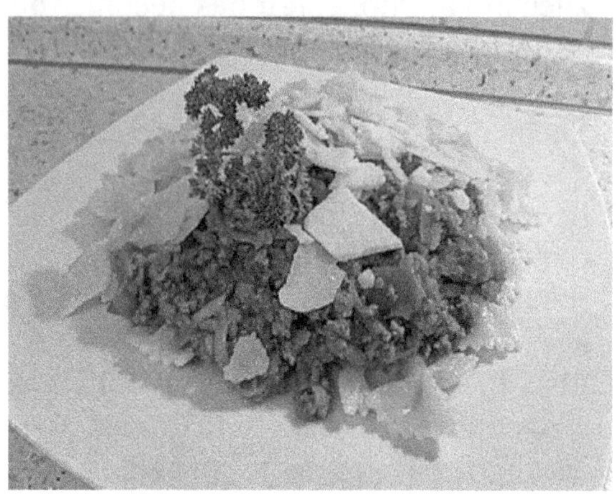

Prep time: 5hrs

One portion

Ingredients

- 2 tbsp oil
- 1kg Minced meat, from beef
- 500g Soup vegetables, (carrot, leek, celery)
- 1 Carrot
- 2 Onion
- 2 Garlic cloves
- One small one Hot peppers, hot
- 50ml red wine, dry
- 800g Tomato (s), from the tin, pieced with juice
- 3 tsp Oregano, dried
- ½ tsp Basil, dried
- 1 Bay leaf

- One pinch sugar
- 250 ml Beef broth, seasoned
- 2 Teaspoons Salt, approx.
- ¼ TL Black pepper
- One teaspoon Beef broth, instant, approx.

Preparation

1. First, in a separate pan, mince the minced meat in the hot oil until it is crumbly. That takes about 10 minutes. Drain the fat, but leave about three tablespoons in the pan. Put the minced meat in the ceramic pot. Now clean the vegetables - carrots, onions, leeks, celery, garlic, and hot peppers - as usual, and, if possible, grate them roughly in a food processor. The vegetable mixture is then gently cooked in the remaining oil over medium heat. Deglaze with a good shot of red wine (but do not boil) and give everything to the minced meat. Finally, add the spices, the dried herbs, and the liquids. Carefully mix and level slightly. Do not be alarmed, the Bolognese seems very plump - but that's the way it should be! The brazing time is approx. 2 hours HIGH and 2 - 3 hours LOW. In between, you may also stir — season with salt, pepper, and a little more brewing powder.
2. Serve with spaghetti and sprinkle with grated hard cheese (e.g., Parmesan).

Vegetables - Lasagna A La Mousse

Vegetarian, without tomatoes - food combining recipe - carbohydrates

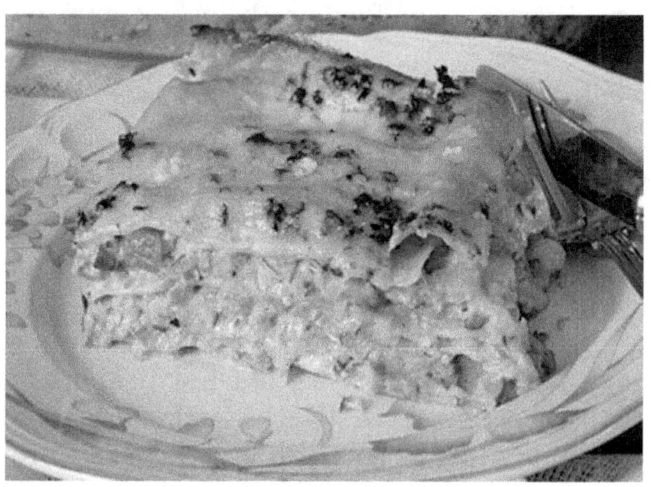

Prep time 5hours

6 portions

Ingredients

- Lasagne plate (s) (without egg - without precooking)
- One big one onion (s), finely diced
- Two toe / n garlic, finely chopped
- 2 m. -Large zucchini, grated
- 2 m. -Large carrot (s), grated
- 1 m. -Large pepper (s), red, small diced
- Two poles/s celery, in fine slices
- 200g mushrooms, in fine slices

- 400g sour cream
- 150g cheese, raw milk Emmentaler, grated
- 1 tbsp olive oil
- salt and pepper
- chili powder
- 400g herbal cream cheese or light herb cream cheese
- Two toe/n garlic, crushed
- Something water
- 100g Parmesan, grated
- Olive oil, for the form

Preparation

1. Heat the olive oil in a large, coated pan (or wok) and fry the onion, garlic, and vegetables vigorously for 5 minutes. Remove the pan/wok from the griddle, allow to cool briefly, and mix in the sour cream and cheese.
2. Mix the herb cream cheese with the garlic and enough water to make a very creamy sauce.
3. Rub a large casserole dish well with olive oil.
4. First, so much cream cheese sauce that the casserole is well covered, then "stratified": a layer of lasagne leaves, cream cheese sauce, a layer of vegetables, a layer of lasagne leaves, cream cheese sauce, vegetables, etc. The last two layers should be lasagna leaves and cream cheese Be sauce.

5. Cover the lasagne with aluminum foil or a lid and leave to soak in the refrigerator for at least 5 hours (better longer, up to 12 hours).
6. Preheat the oven to 180 degrees top/bottom heat.
7. Sprinkle the grated Parmesan cheese over the lasagna and bake for 45 minutes.

Tips:

- Raw milk cheese (e.g., Emmentaler) - no matter what fat level - counts among the Haysche food combining (as well as Parmesan) to the neutral group. That it is raw milk cheese must be noted on the packaging or necessarily ask when buying at the cheese counter.
- If the Emmentaler is made from pasteurized milk, it belongs to the protein group and is not suitable for this dish.

Fried Noodles With Vegetables And Meat (Asian)

3 portions

Prep time: 20 mins

Ingredients

- 200g Chinese egg noodles
- 2 liters water
- 1 tbsp salt
- 2 tbsp oil
- 200g pork or turkey meat
- 3 spring onions
- 1 Pepper
- 2 Carrot
- ¼ liters of water, hot
- One teaspoon of broth, grained
- 2 tbsp soy sauce
- 1 tbsp cornstarch
- Salt and pepper
- 2 tbsp oil
- Soy sauce

preparation

1. Boil, the boiling noodles, salted water by the Preparations for packing and strain.
2. Fry the meat in a large pan with oil for 3 minutes.
3. Clean the spring onions, wash and cut into 2 cm long pieces. Wash the peppers, cut in

half, corer them, and cut into strips. Wash the carrots, peel, and grate or cut into thin slices.

4. Add the sliced vegetables to the meat in the pan and fry for 2 minutes.
5. Mix the stock, soy sauce, and cornstarch well in a bowl, add to the frying pan and add to the rest of the ingredients.
6. Heat the oil in another pan, add the drained noodles and cook for about 3 minutes. Then add the vegetable-meat mixture and mix.
7. Put in a preheated bowl.

Salmon With Vegetables And Potatoes

Prep time: 30 mins

4 portions

Ingredients

- 1 Salmon (wild salmon, in whole)
- 6 m. -Large potato
- 4 m. -Large carrot
- Two broccoli
- 4 m. -Large tomatoes
- ¼ liters of vegetable stock
- 1 cup cream
- 2 tbsp herbs, French (or of your choice), chopped
- Butter, cut into flakes
- Salt and pepper

preparation

1. Peel the potatoes and carrots. Divide the broccoli into florets. Halve the potatoes and cut the carrots into 3 - 5 cm long pieces.
2. Cook the potatoes and carrots for about 10 minutes and the broccoli in salted water for about 3 minutes. Drain the water and distribute the potatoes and vegetables on the meat pan from the oven. Divide the salmon into about eight portions and place between vegetables and potatoes. Wash the tomatoes, cut crosswise, and also put on the

tin. Now mix the broth and cream with the herbs, salt, and pepper (Tip: If you love garlic, you can also add it to the broth). Now pour this broth over the ingredients on the plate and spread butter flakes over the vegetables and salmon as needed.

3. Cook in a preheated oven at 200 ° C, circulating air for approx. 30 minutes. Serve hot.

4. The recipe can also be prepared well for a party and - when it's time - put it in the oven.

Fried Salmon On Mediterranean Vegetables

Prep time: 35 mins

4 portions

Ingredients

- 4 Pepper (s), red, coarsely crushed
- 1 m. -Large eggplant (s), roughly minced
- 3 m. -Large zucchini, roughly minced
- One bunch vegetable onion (s), roughly chopped
- 750g Salmon fillet (s) (TK), thawed, pieced
- 1 Lemon (s), the juice of it
- One glass Pesto (basil pesto)
- Flour
- Seasoned Salt
- Olive oil
- Vegetable stock
- Ketchup (curry ketchup), spicy
- Paprika
- Pepper
- One pinch of sugar
- Fat for the mold

Preparation

1. Fry the prepared vegetables in a large pan while stirring with the hot olive oil. Add a little vegetable stock and let it simmer for about 7-10 minutes with the lid. Season

with curry ketchup, herbal salt, paprika, pepper, and sugar as needed.

2. In the meantime, marinate the thawed salmon pieces with lemon juice and then season with herb salt. Turn in a little flour and brown on both sides in olive oil.

3. Put the vegetables in a greased casserole dish, arrange the salmon pieces on top, and spread generously with the basil pesto.

4. In the preheated oven overcool at 200 ° C convection for about 7-10 minutes.

5. This tastes baguette or flatbread.

Oven Chicken With Vegetables

Quick recipe with chicken thighs on carrots and potatoes

4 portions

Prep time: 1hrs

Ingredients

- 4 Chicken legs, fresh or frozen
- 5 Potato
- 5 Carrot
- Two toe garlic, roughly chopped
- Onion
- 100 ml olive oil
- One teaspoon of paprika powder, sweet
- One teaspoon of paprika powder, pink
- One teaspoon of salt
- One teaspoon of thyme
- Three toe/n Garlic, pressed

Preparation

1. Peel and dice the potatoes and carrots. Peel and halve the onion, finely dice one half and cut the other into rings. Add together with two coarsely chopped garlic cloves to the potato and carrot cubes.
2. Then mix a marinade with oil, paprika, salt, thyme, and pressed garlic. So that the chicken thighs brush (very important: also

marinade under the skin!). Add the rest of the marinade to 1 - 2 teaspoons of the potato and carrot mixture and mix well, season with salt, if necessary.

3. Put the vegetable mixture into a large baking dish, put the chicken thighs on top, and bake at 200 ° C for 60 - 70 minutes. Possibly. Brush with remaining marinade. After about half of the baking time, I turn the thighs and let them take some color from below for a few minutes. To make the skin crispy, but in any case, turn it again a few minutes before the end of cooking time.

4. Vegetables and meat become very fragrant when they are baked together, and after the Schnipper, the whole thing cooks itself by itself. With certainty, the recipe can also be changed with other vegetables (zucchini, paprika, ...) or other spices.

Beefsteak With Mustard And Herb Topping And Vegetables

Prep time: 3 hrs 10mins

2 portions

Ingredients

- Two thick Beefsteak (s) (beef steaks), each about 250 g, well-hung
- 3 m. -Large carrot
- 2 m. -Large zucchini
- 2 TL heaped Mustard medium hot
- Something herbs of Provence
- Something pepper
- Something salt or Himalayan salt
- Something olive oil or coconut oil
- Herbs, fresh (thyme, garlic, mushroom)
- Something Leeks or onions, optional

preparation

1. Rub the two steaks well with olive oil and cover for at least 3 hours in the fridge (better already one day before). Half an hour before frying (preferably in an iron pan), take out of the refrigerator — Preheat the oven to 80 ° C without circulating air.
2. Make the pan very hot and fry the steaks without further oil. Fry for 1.5 - 2 (otherwise 3) minutes on each side, depending on the thickness.

3. Sprinkle the steaks with mustard, sprinkle with Provence pepper and herbs, wrap in aluminum foil, and place in the oven. Let rest for 10-15 minutes. The steaks are salted after resting.

4. In the meantime, peel the carrots, wash the zucchini, and cut both into small pieces. Fry in a pan with two tablespoons of coconut oil (if necessary, sauté onions and leeks) and let it cook. Season with salt, pepper, and fresh herbs to taste.

CHAPTER 15

POULTRY RECIPES

Basque Chicken

For: 4 people

Prep time: 60 mins

Ingredients

- One whole chicken about 1.4 or 1.5 kg
- 1 kg of tomatoes
- One red
- 1 yellow pepper
- 200 g mushrooms
- One onion
- One clove of garlic
- 1 tbsp. Oil
- Two glasses dry white wine
- 2 tbsp. Flour
- 1/2 tsp. Coffee of Espelette
- Salt and pepper from the mill

Preparation

1. Boil some water in a saucepan and immerse the tomatoes in it for 30 seconds. Peel them, seed them, and cut them in eight. Wash the mushrooms and cut them in half. Wash the peppers and cut them into thin strips. Peel the onions and garlic and chop them.
2. Cut the chicken into eight pieces.

3. Heat the oil in the casserole. Brown the onions and garlic and add the chicken pieces for about 10 minutes.
4. Sprinkle the flour on the chicken pieces. Add tomato pieces, mushrooms, pepper strips, chili, and white wine — season and cook in the covered casserole for 40 minutes.
5. Serve in a hollow dish with the chicken pieces on it.

Nutrition Facts

Serving Size:1

Amount for Serving

Calories from Fat 135

Calories 470

% Daily Value*

- 23% Total Fat 15g grams
- 18% Saturated Fat 3.5g grams
- Trans Fat 0g grams
- 30% Cholesterol 90mg milligrams
- 70% Sodium 1690mg milligrams
- 16% Total Carbohydrates 47g grams
- 20% Dietary Fiber 5g grams
- Sugars 8g grams
- Protein 35g grams

* Percent Daily Values are based on a 2000 calorie diet.

Blue Corded Chicken Breast

Prep time: 25 mins

4 people

Ingredients

- 4 chicken breasts
- 2 slices of ham
- 4 slices of Comté cheese
- 100g of bread crumbs
- 2 eggs
- 40g of butter
- Salt and pepper from the grinder

Preparing

1. Cut the chicken fillets in their thickness, leaving the two parts attached. Place half a slice of ham on one side. Place a good slice of county cheese and close the chicken cutlet. On a plate, beat two eggs with a fork to make an omelet. On another plate, pour bread crumbs. Dip the chicken breast with the ham and cheese on the plate with the eggs and dip in the bread crumbs. Bread crumbs will stick on the escape thanks to the eggs. Let the blue strips cook in the pan in the butter for 4 to 5 minutes on each side.

Nutrition Facts

Serving Size grams (136 g)

Serving for 1

Calories 120 cal

Calories from Fat 0.00

Amount Per Serving % DV

- Total Fat 1.5 g 2 %
- Saturated Fat 0.5 g
- Trans. Fat 0.0 g
- Polyunsaturated Fat 0.3 g
- Omega 3 0 mg
- EPA 0.00 mg
- DHA 0.00 mg
- Monounsaturated Fat 0.5 g
- Cholesterol 70 mg
- Sodium 520 mg 22 %

Amount Per Serving % DV

- Total Carbohydrate 0 g 0 %
- Dietary Fiber 0 g 0 %
- Sugars 0 g
- Other Carbohydrate 0.00 g
- Protein 27 g
- Potassium 380 mg 11 %
- Niacin 60 %
- Vitamin B6 25 %

- Vitamin B12

Hunter Chicken

Prep time: 60 mins

4 people

Ingredients

- One whole chicken about 1.4 or 1.5 kg
- 300 g mushrooms
- Three shallots
- One bouquet garni
- 10 cl. White wine
- 30 cl. Veal stock
- 20 cl. Of fresh cream
- One bunch of tarragon
- Three sprigs of parsley
- 1 tbsp. Flour
- Six potatoes
- 20 g. Butter
- 1 tbsp. Tablespoons
- Salt and pepper from the mill

Preparation

1. Peel the shallots and chop them. Cut the mushrooms in four.
2. Cut the chicken into eight pieces.
3. In a casserole, melt the butter with the oil and fry the pieces of chicken. Add shallots and mushrooms and fry for 5 minutes.
4. Add the flour, moisten with the white wine. Add the veal stock, the bouquet garni, and

the potatoes. Season. Cover and cook for 30 minutes. Finally, add the liquid cream and cook another 10 minutes.

5. Serve with parsley and chopped tarragon on top.

Nutrition Facts

Serving Size: 1 serving

Amount for Serving

- Calories 606.4
- Total Fat 44.6 g
- Saturated Fat 26.3 g
- Polyunsaturated Fat 2.0 g
- Monounsaturated Fat 13.8 g
- Cholesterol 170.6 mg
- Sodium 950.0 mg
- Potassium 353.3 mg
- Total Carbohydrate 1.5 g
- Dietary Fiber 0.0 g
- Sugars 0.0 g
- Protein 48.4 g
- Vitamin (A) 24.2 %
- Vitamin (B 12) 23.8 %
- Vitamin (B-6) 25.4 %
- Vitamin (C) 1.4 %
- Vitamin (D) 3.4 %
- Vitamin (E) 2.8 %
- Calcium 82.4 %
- Copper 4.3 %

- Folate 6.0 %
- Iron 8.2 %
- Magnesium 13.6 %
- Manganese 1.5 %
- Niacin 44.8 %
- Pantothenic Acid 11.8 %
- Phosphorus 76.0 %
- Riboflavin 30.9 %
- Selenium 45.0 %
- Thiamin 11.2 %
- Zinc 30.0 %

The amount of daily values is based on a diet of 2,000 calories. Depending on your calorie needs, your daily values can be higher or lower.

Duck Breast With Figs And Vinegar

Prep time: 60 mins

Six portions

Ingredients

- Three duck breasts (or fillets) of 350 g each
- 18 fresh figs
- Two apples
- 10 cl of sherry vinegar
- 1 tbsp. Liquid honey
- 30 gr butter
- 1 tbsp. Coffeeberry roses
- One sprig of rosemary
- Salt and freshly ground pepper

Preparation

1. Heat a non-stick frying pan. When it is hot, put the breasts in, skin side below. Turn the heat down to low and cook for 15 to 20 minutes, removing the fat from time to time and without turning the breasts.
2. Meanwhile, wash and empty the apples. Cut them into thick slices. Melt the butter in a pan and brown the slices of apples. Put them on paper towels.
3. Melt the honey in a frying pan, put the figs on them, and cook for 10 minutes, turning them gently so that they are well coated with honey. Take them out of the pan and

pour the vinegar. Cook for a minute over high heat, stirring with a wooden spatula.

4. Cut the duck breasts into slices and place them in the hot plates. Add salt and pepper. Add the slices of apples and put the figs on top. Sprinkle with honey sauce and vinegar.
5. Sprinkle with pink berries and rosemary and serve immediately.

Nutrition Facts

Amount Per Serving (2 servings)

Calories 320 Calories from Fat 54

% Daily Value*

- Total Fat 6g 9%
- Saturated Fat 1g 5%
- Cholesterol 89mg 30%
- Sodium 178mg 7%
- Potassium 735mg 21%
- Total Carbohydrates 29g 10%
- Dietary Fiber 3g 12%
- Sugars 22g
- Protein 25g 50%
- Vitamin A 4%
- Vitamin C 12.2%
- Calcium 3.5%
- Iron 33.7%

* Percent Daily Values are based on a 2000 calorie diet.

Duck Breast With Mirabelle Plums

Prep time: 30 mins

4 portions

Ingredients

- Two duck breast (or fillet) approximately 350 g each
- 300 g frozen Mirabelle plums (or fresh)
- 1 tsp. Chicken, ground coffee
- 3 cl of plum brandy
- 50 g of cold butter
- Salt and pepper from the mill

Preparation

1. Let the Mirabelle thaw at room temperature.
2. Remove some fat from the sides of the breasts. Cut the skin in crosspieces, using a sharp knife. Put them skin side in a hot pan, without adding fat. Cook for 6 minutes on high heat, turn them over and cook for 4 minutes. Let them rest on a plate covered with aluminum foil.
3. Empty the grease from the pan without wiping it. Throw in Mirabelle plums and cook for 2 to 3 minutes while stirring. Remove them from the pan and keep them warm. Replace with the bottom of poultry diluted in water and the brandy. Bring to

the boil by peeling off the cooking juices with a wooden spoon. Stir in small pieces of butter while whisking.

4. Slice the duck breasts. Stir the juice in the sauce. Mix.

5. Arrange the slices of filleted duck on the plates, pour the sauce and add the mirabelles. Serve immediately.

Nutrition Facts

Calories help 102   (427 kJ)

Calories from fat help 32

% Daily Value 1

- Total Fat help 3.5g 5%
- Sat. Fat help 1.1g 5%
- Cholesterol help 64mg 21%
- Sodium 47mg 2%
- Total Carbs. Help 0g 0%
- Dietary Fiber help 0g 0%
- Protein help 16.5g
- Calcium help 2.5mg
- Potassium 222.4mg

Duck Leg Confit With Turnips

Prep time: 80 mins

Six people

Ingredients

- Six duck legs with skin
- 90 g butter
- One bay leaf
- Three sprigs rosemary
- Five peppercorns
- 1 tbsp.
- 1 cup coriander beans one chicken stock cube
- 1 kg small turnips
- 1 tbsp. Sugar-shaved soup
- Oil
- Salt and freshly ground pepper

Preparation

1. Heat a cast-iron casserole with a drizzle of oil, melt 30 g butter, and put the duck legs to brown on both sides over low heat without drilling.
2. When the legs are golden brown on both sides, put them all back in the pan; salt, add the bay leaf and a sprig of rosemary, pepper and cilantro seeds and crumble the chicken broth and pour a large glass of water; cover and let simmer for 45 minutes over low

heat by turning the thighs regularly and adding water if necessary.

3. Meanwhile, peel the turnips and cut them into thick slices. Put them in a saucepan, add salt, pepper, powder with sugar, add the remaining butter in parcels and cover with water; cook over very low heat until all the liquid has evaporated, then reserve covered.

4. When the duck legs are cooked, put the sauté pan back on high heat and sauté the turnips 3 min until they begin to caramelize.

5. Serve warm, duck legs with turnips.

Nutrition Facts

Servings Per Recipe: 1

Serving Size: 1 serving

Amount Per Serving

- Calories 314.6
- Total Fat 23.3 g
- Saturated Fat 7.0 g
- Polyunsaturated Fat 3.4 g
- Monounsaturated Fat 11.5 g
- Cholesterol 117.9 mg
- Sodium 101.2 mg
- Potassium 0.0 mg
- Total Carbohydrate 0.0 g
- Dietary Fiber 0.0 g

- Sugars 0.0 g
- Protein 24.6 g
- Vitamin (A) 0.0 %
- Vitamin (B-12) 0.0 %
- Vitamin (B-6) 0.0 %
- Vitamin (C) 2.3 %
- Vitamin (D) 0.0 %
- Vitamin (E) 0.0 %
- Calcium 0.9 %
- Copper 0.0 %
- Folate 0.0 %
- Iron 10.6 %
- Magnesium 0.0 %
- Manganese 0.0 %
- Niacin 26.5 %
- Pantothenic Acid 0.0 %
- Phosphorus 0.0 %
- Riboflavin 0.0 %
- Selenium 28.7 %
- Thiamin 0.0 %
- Zinc 0.0 %

*Percent Daily Values are based on a 2,000 calories diet. Your daily values may be higher or lower depending on your calorie needs.

Duck With Orange In A Casserole

Prep time: 90 mins

4 people

Ingredients

- 4 duck legs
- 3 oranges
- One lemon
- 2 tbsp. coffee, sugar
- 2 tbsp. vinegar
- Olive oil
- Salt and freshly ground pepper

Preparation

1. Heat the bottom of olive oil over high heat in a casserole. Put the duck legs to brown in the pan for 10 minutes, turning on each side. When they are golden brown, salt, pepper, lower the heat, and cover the pan for 1 hour of cooking.
2. Cut the oranges to extract the quarters. Put the orange quarters in the pan for the last 20 minutes of cooking.
3. After cooking, extract the legs and orange quarters of the casserole. Set aside the cooking juices as well.
4. To deglaze and caramelize, add the vinegar into the bottom of the casserole with the sugar. Squeeze the lemon and pour in the

saucepan the juice and set aside the cooking juices.

5. Serve the duck legs surrounded by wedges of orange and brush with the sauce.

Nutrition Facts

Servings Per Recipe: 12

Serving Size: 1 serving

Amount for Serving

- Calories 467.4
- Total Fat 23.7 g
- Saturated Fat 6.9 g
- Polyunsaturated Fat 3.7 g
- Monounsaturated Fat 11.3 g
- Cholesterol 221.1 mg
- Sodium 237.5 mg
- Potassium 81.5 mg
- Total Carbohydrate 6.4 g
- Dietary Fiber 0.8 g
- Sugars 2.3 g
- Protein 51.4 g
- Vitamin (A) 2.9 %
- Vitamin (B-12) 0.0 %
- Vitamin (B-6) 1.6 %
- Vitamin (C) 32.1 %
- Vitamin (D) 0.0 %
- Vitamin (E) 0.6 %
- Calcium 3.3 %
- Copper 1.3 %

- Folate 2.6 %
- Iron 22.4 %
- Magnesium 1.2 %
- Manganese 0.8 %
- Niacin 56.5 %
- Pantothenic Acid 0.8 %
- Phosphorus 1.1 %
- Riboflavin 1.8 %
- Selenium 59.7 %
- Thiamin 2.3 %
- Zinc 0.4 %

The amount of daily values is based on a diet of 2,000 calories. Depending on your calorie needs, your daily values can be higher or lower.

Rabbit Recipe With Mustard And Mushrooms

Prep time: 90 mins

4 people

Ingredients

- One saddle and two rabbit thighs
- 2 tbsp. olive oil
- 40 g butter
- 1 tbsp. flour
- 15 cl of cider
- Two sprigs of thyme
- Two sprigs of rosemary
- One bay leaf
- 600 g mushrooms
- 600 g mushrooms
- Two shallots
- 3 tbsp. old-fashioned mustard
- 2 tbsp. Dijon mustard
- 30 cl liquid cream
- Salt and freshly ground pepper

Preparation

1. Heat the oil and 40 g of butter in a pan and put the rabbit pieces to color on all sides. Salt, pepper, powder with flour and mix. Then pour the cider, add the sprigs of thyme, rosemary and bay leaf, cover and let simmer for 45 minutes over low heat, stirring regularly.

2. Cut the hard and earthy part of the mushrooms' feet, clean them and slice them. Peel and mince the shallots; Wash, dry, and chop the parsley.
3. In a frying pan, froth 40 g butter and sauté the mushrooms for 5 minutes over high heat. At the end of the cooking, add the minced shallots and parsley, salt, pepper, and mix.
4. Mix the two mustards in a bowl with the cream, then pour this mixture into the casserole; add the mushrooms, mix slightly and let simmer 20 min again, without covering and over low heat.
5. Serve with fresh pasta.

Nutritional Information

Serving

- Energy (kcal) 487 kcal
- Energy (kJ) 2036 kJ
- Protein (g) 11.9 g
- Carbohydrate incl. fiber (g) 71.0 g
- Carbohydrate excl. fiber (g) 68.2 g
- Sugar (g) 4.4 g
- Fiber (g) 2.8 g
- Fat (g) 16.2 g
- Saturated fat (g) 3.9 g
- Unsaturated fat (g) 10.6 g
- Monounsaturated fat (g) 5.0 g
- Polyunsaturated fat (g) 0.7 g
- Trans fat (g) 0.1 g

- Cholesterol (mg) 0 mg
- Sodium (mg) 406 mg
- Salt (g) 1.01 g
- Vitamin A (IU) 41 IU
- Vitamin C (mg) 4.7 mg
- Calcium (mg) 9 mg
- Iron (mg) 0.35 mg
- Potassium (mg) 135 mg

Mushroom And Tarragon Rabbit

Prep time: 90 mins

6 people

Ingredients

- 1 rabbit rasp of 300 g
- 2 rabbit legs of 450 g in total
- 50 cl of beer
- 3 shallots
- 1 cubic broth
- 3 tarragon stalks
- 200 gr mushrooms
- 60 gr butter
- 2 tablespoons of flour
- 2 teaspoons of starch (corn starch)
- 1 lemon yellow
- 1 teaspoon of caster sugar
- Salt and freshly ground pepper

Preparation

1. Flour, salt, and pepper the rabbit bits. Make them come back with the butter in a casserole.
2. Squeeze the lemon juice. Slice the shallots. Melt the cube broth in a glass of boiling water. Pour the beer into the casserole, add the sugar, the shallots, and the lemon juice. Pour the broth to cover the pieces. Bring to

a boil, lower heat, cover, and cook gently for 1 hour.

3. Wash the tarragon, clean it, and rinse it. Peel the mushrooms and slice them. Add them to the casserole and continue cooking for 30 minutes. Put the rabbit pieces in a serving dish.

4. Mix 2 teaspoons of cornflour in a tablespoon of water. Pour this mixture into the casserole, cook, stirring over high heat to thicken the sauce. Correct the seasoning, pour over the rabbit. Decorate with tarragon leaves.

Nutrition Facts

Serving Size: 1 serving

Amount for Serving

- Calories 246.6
- Total Fat 6.4 g
- Saturated Fat 1.2 g
- Polyunsaturated Fat 0.8 g
- Monounsaturated Fat 3.8 g
- Cholesterol 61.2 mg
- Sodium 165.6 mg
- Potassium 254.2 mg
- Total Carbohydrate 20.4 g
- Dietary Fiber 2.9 g
- Sugars 0.9 g
- Protein 20.1 g
- Vitamin A 113.3 %

- Vitamin (B-12) 0.2 %
- Vitamin (B-6) 4.1 %
- Vitamin (C) 10.1 %
- Vitamin (D) 4.4 %
- Vitamin (E) 3.3 %
- Calcium 3.1 %
- Copper 6.1 %
- Folate 5.5 %
- Iron 6.2 %
- Magnesium 3.8 %
- Manganese 13.0 %
- Niacin 6.8 %
- Pantothenic Acid 4.7 %
- Phosphorus 4.6 %
- Riboflavin 7.4 %
- Selenium 3.9 %
- Thiamin 3.0 %
- Zinc 1.8 %

* Regular percentages are based on a diet of 2,000 calories. Based on your calorie requirements, your regular values may be higher or lower.

Gibelotte Of Rabbit In A Casserole

Prep time: 90 mins

6 portions

Ingredients

- One rabbit sirloin 300g
- Two rabbit thighs 220g each
- 200g breast half salt
- Six parsnips
- Four onions
- Six cloves garlic
- One bouquet garni
- 75cl white wine type chardonnay
- 15cl red port
- 5cl marc burgundy
- 1 tbsp. old-fashioned mustard
- 1 tbsp. tablespoon flour
- olive oil
- salt and freshly ground pepper

Preparation

1. Peel and chop the onions. Peel the parsnips and cut them into four.
2. Cut the breast into bacon. Brown the rabbit with bacon, garlic, and onions in a casserole. Brown all, then flour.
3. Flambé with the marc de Bourgogne. Deglaze with the port and pour the white wine into the casserole.

4. Add the bouquet garni and season. After 30 minutes, put the parsnips in the pan and cook for another 30 minutes. Add the mustard for the last 5 minutes of cooking and stir to bind.

Nutrition Facts

Serving Size: 1 serving

Amount for Serving

- Calories 272.0
- Total Fat 5.6 g
- Saturated Fat 1.9 g
- Polyunsaturated Fat 1.0 g
- Monounsaturated Fat 1.5 g
- Cholesterol 157.0 mg
- Sodium 150.7 mg
- Potassium 657.9 mg
- Total Carbohydrate 10.4 g
- Dietary Fiber 0.9 g
- Sugars 1.4 g
- Protein 43.6 g
- Vitamin (A) 8.7 %
- Vitamin (B-12) 137.2 %
- Vitamin (B-6) 31.6 %
- Vitamin (C) 9.6 %
- Vitamin (D) 0.0 %
- Vitamin (E) 6.2 %
- Calcium 8.8 %
- Copper 15.8 %

- Folate 7.2 %
- Iron 40.5 %
- Magnesium 14.1 %
- Manganese 15.5 %
- Niacin 41.5 %
- Pantothenic Acid 2.8 %
- Phosphorus 35.7 %
- Riboflavin 9.3 %
- Selenium 30.1 %
- Thiamin 4.8 %
- Zinc 23.1 %

Regular percentages are based on a diet of 2,000 calories. Based on your calorie requirements, your regular values may be higher or lower.

CONCLUSION

MISTAKES TO AVOID

Starting to eat Keto is rather simple once you understand the basic principles (focus on good fats, limit carbohydrates, and moderate proteins). However, there are a few beginner's mistakes to avoid, so be aware of them from the start!

The Seven Mistakes To Avoid:

1 / Succumb To The Call Of Sugar The First Days

At first, we go through the delicate phase of entering ketosis, and cravings for sweets can manifest themselves with great force. Eating snacks rich in lipids (pâté and pickle, avocado, olives, or "fatty sweets") helps to pass this course. Certain foods (generally industrial) are both rich in lipids and carbohydrates (crisps, pastries). They are to be avoided completely of course, especially since their lipids are generally very toxic (trans fat).

2 / Make Small Deviations Which Cause The Loss Of The State Of Ketosis

Subsequently, the sweet cravings disappear in most "ketones," but some temporarily lose the state of ketosis by cracking on a croissant, some cookies or even fruit or bread. The consequences can either be a plateau in weight loss, which is not dramatic, or a return to the symptoms of adaptation, with headache, nausea, body aches, sore throat. Personally, I have not cracked once since the adoption of this lifestyle. I find enough pleasure in my meals, my seed bread and my "keto" desserts and never again feel the need to succumb to anything that would make me lose this pleasant state.

3 / Eat Too Little Fat

Fats, especially saturated fats (butter, cream, cheese, meat), have suffered such discredit in recent decades that it is difficult to imagine that not really, eating fat does not make you fat (like eating cucumbers does not make you green). The storage of energy in fat cells takes place in the liver under the effect of insulin. With a very low production of this hormone, as by this food mode, we do not store but on the contrary, burns our provisions.

And finding the sensations of lipids is rather pleasant: spinach is much better with cream or butter! I thought I would hate cottage cheese because I had imposed myself with 0% cottage cheese in the past, which gives the feeling of eating plaster. Since I rediscovered 40% Fromage blanc, with homemade whipped cream, it has been one of my favorite desserts!

4 / Exaggerate Your Consumption Of Dairy Products Or Nuts

If white cheese contains good saturated fat, it also contains, like cream and nuts, a certain amount of carbohydrates. The desserts that we make from nuts, almonds, and dairy products are so delicious that it is tempting to exceed your hunger. Some people realize that reducing or even stopping the consumption of dairy products and nuts helps them to overcome a plateau.

5 / Having Unrealistic Expectations

This diet generally brings countless benefits, and weight loss is one of them. But it is rarely linear. Personally, I lost 5 kg in the first 15 days; then, I did not lose any more for 4 months, then I lost another 4 kg in one month. Since then, my weight has remained stable. I would still like to lose 2 or 3 kg but at the same time, I no longer focus on the scale. I carry over the size 38 of my youth, and especially feel so good that the balance is secondary. Hoping for too fast or too unrealistic results can be disheartening.

6 / To Restrict Oneself Too Much Or Not To Vary The Menus Enough

The keto diet is not a temporary diet that we follow a few weeks to lose pounds before summer. Once we have understood, reached and experienced it, we continue it! I have read testimonials from people who have been in ketosis for 10 or 20 years, and who enjoy optimal health and low, consistent body weight. But to appreciate this way of life, you have to find pleasures, vary the dishes and constantly discover new ways to accommodate them. Of course, we each have our preferences. Personally, I particularly like anchovies, eggs and chocolate. I eat it several times a week, but I also vary with other foods and enjoy successful discoveries (I also sometimes feel sorry for completely failed attempts!). Find the color of the different vegetables,

7 / Drink Too Much Alcohol.

The alcohol in a measured quantity is not incompatible with the Keto diet mode. Some alcohols contain few carbohydrates, such as vodka, whiskey, gin. Added with sparkling water, a dash of lemon and fresh mint, they can be an occasional aperitif. Some wines are lower in carbohydrates than others (champagne only contains one gram of carbohydrate per glass, dry wines contain 3.5 gr). On the other hand, beer is really very rich in carbohydrates. If alcohol does not cause ketosis to be lost in most people, it metabolizes before the rest.

www.ingramcontent.com/pod-product-compliance
Lightning Source LLC
Chambersburg PA
CBHW071604030726
47593CB00001BA/315